# The Changing Landscape of Urologic Practice

*Editor*

DEEPAK A. KAPOOR

# UROLOGIC CLINICS
# OF NORTH AMERICA

www.urologic.theclinics.com

*Editor-In-Chief*
KEVIN R. LOUGHLIN

May 2021 • Volume 48 • Number 2

**ELSEVIER**

1600 John F. Kennedy Boulevard • Suite 1800 • Philadelphia, Pennsylvania, 19103-2899

http://www.theclinics.com

**UROLOGIC CLINICS OF NORTH AMERICA Volume 48, Number 2**
**May 2021 ISSN 0094-0143, ISBN-13: 978-0-323-79064-2**

Editor: Kerry Holland
Developmental Editor: Diana Ang

*Urologic Clinics of North America* (ISSN 0094-0143) is published quarterly by Elsevier Inc., 360 Park Avenue South, New York, NY 10010-1710. Months of issue are February, May, August, and November. Business and Editorial Offices: 1600 John F. Kennedy Blvd., Suite 1800, Philadelphia, PA 19103-2899. Periodicals postage paid at New York, NY and additional mailing offices. Subscription prices are $395.00 per year (US individuals), $1033.00 per year (US institutions), $100.00 per year (US students and residents), $450.00 per year (Canadian individuals), $1059.00 per year (Canadian institutions), $100.00 per year (Canadian students/residents), $520.00 per year (foreign individuals), $1059.00 per year (foreign institutions), and $240.00 per year (foreign students/residents). Foreign air speed delivery is included in all *Clinics* subscription prices. All prices are subject to change without notice. **POSTMASTER:** Send address changes to *Urologic Clinics of North America*, Elsevier Health Sciences Division, Subscription Customer Service, 3251 Riverport Lane, Maryland Heights, MO 63043. **Customer Service: 1-800-654-2452 (US). From outside the United States, call 1-314-447-8871. Fax: 1-314-447-8029. E-mail: JournalsCustomerServiceusa@elsevier.com (for print support) and JournalsOnlineSupport-usa@elsevier.com (for online support).**

*Reprints.* For copies of 100 or more, of articles in this publication, please contact the Commercial Reprints Department, Elsevier Inc., 360 Park Avenue South, New York, New York 10010-1710. Tel.: 212-633-3874; Fax: 212-633-3820; E-mail: reprints@elsevier.com.

*Urologic Clinics of North America* is covered in MEDLINE/PubMed (*Index Medicus*), *Excerpta Medica, Current Contents/Clinical Medicine, Science Citation Index,* and *ISI/BIOMED.*

# Contributors

## EDITOR-IN-CHIEF

**KEVIN R. LOUGHLIN, MD, MBA**
Emeritus Professor of Surgery (Urology),
Harvard Medical School, Visiting Scientist,
Vascular Biology Research Program at Boston
Children's Hospital, Boston, Massachusetts

## EDITOR

**DEEPAK A. KAPOOR, MD**
Market President, Integrated Medical
Professionals, PLLC, Chairman and Chief
Ecosystem Officer, Solaris Health Holdings,
LLC, Clinical Professor of Urology, Icahn
School of Medicine at Mount Sinai,
Farmingdale, New York

## AUTHORS

**KARI BAILEY, MD**
Partner, AAUrology, PA, Annapolis, Maryland

**MICHAEL COOKSON, MD, FACS**
Chairman, Department of Urology, University
of Oklahoma, Oklahoma City, Oklahoma

**LAURA CROCITTO, MD, MHA**
Chief Medical Officer/Vice President, Cancer
Services, Professor of Urology, UCSF
Medical Center, Helen Diller Family
Comprehensive Cancer Center, San
Francisco, California

**RYAN DORNBIER, MD**
Department of Urology, Stritch School of
Medicine, Loyola University Medical Center,
Maywood, Illinois

**MATTHEW GETTMAN, MD**
Professor, Mayo Clinic, Rochester, Minnesota

**EVAN R. GOLDFISCHER, MD, MBA, CPE,
CPI**
Director of Research, Urology Division, Premier
Medical Group, Clinical Assistant Professor of
Urology, New York Medical College

**CHRISTOPHER M. GONZALEZ, MD, MBA**
Department of Urology, Stritch School of
Medicine, Loyola University Medical Center,
Maywood, Illinois

**JASON HAFRON, MD**
Associate Professor of Urology, William
Beaumont School of Medicine, Director of
Robotic Surgery, Beaumont Health, Director
of Clinical Research, Michigan Institute of
Urology, Troy, Michigan

**MARA R. HOLTON, MD**
Managing Partner, AAUrology, PA, Annapolis,
Maryland

**DEEPAK A. KAPOOR, MD**
Market President, Integrated Medical
Professionals, PLLC, Chairman and Chief
Ecosystem Officer, Solaris Health Holdings,
LLC, Clinical Professor of Urology, Icahn
School of Medicine at Mount Sinai,
Farmingdale, New York

**GARY M. KIRSH, MD**
Market President, The Urology Group
Cincinnati, President, Solaris Health Holdings,
Cincinnati, Ohio

**ERIC KIRSHENBAUM, MD**
UroPartners, Grayslake, Illinois

**KATHLEEN L. LATINO, MD, FACS**
Chief Medical Officer, Solaris Health Partners,
Medical Director, Integrated Medical
Professionals, Farmingdale, New York

**KEVIN R. LOUGHLIN, MD, MBA**
Emeritus Professor of Surgery (Urology),
Harvard Medical School, Visiting Scientist,
Vascular Biology Research Program at Boston
Children's Hospital, Boston, Massachusetts

**JENNIFER NAUHEIM, MD**
Resident, Department of Urology, Montefiore
Medical Center, Bronx, New York

**AMANDA C. NORTH, MD**
Associate Professor, Department of
Urology, Montefiore Medical Center, Bronx,
New York

**JAKE QUARLES**
Michigan Institute of Urology, Troy, Michigan

**THOMAS H. RECHTSCHAFFEN, MD, FACS**
Integrated Medical Professionals, PLLC,
Farmingdale, New York

**EUGENE Y. RHEE, MD, MBA**
Regional Chief of Urology, Southern California
Kaiser Permanente, San Diego, California;
National Chair, Urology, Permanente
Federation

**CAITLIN SHEPHERD, MD**
Urologic Oncology Fellow, University of
Oklahoma, Oklahoma City, Oklahoma

**NEAL SHORE, MD, FACS**
Director, CPI, Carolina Research Center,
Myrtle Beach, South Carolina

**AARON SPITZ, MD**
Orange County Urology, Irvine, California

**CHRISTOPHER G. STAPPAS, J.D, CFP**
Private Wealth Advisor, Summit Financial, LLC,
Parsippany, New Jersey

# Contents

**Foreword: Between the Forty-Yard Lines: Health Care Reform and its Impact on the Changing Landscape of Urologic Practice**     xi

Kevin R. Loughlin

**Preface: Embracing Change in Urologic Practice: Both Without and Within**     xv

Deepak A. Kapoor

**Workforce Issues in Urology**     161

Ryan Dornbier and Christopher M. Gonzalez

> The future supply of urologists is not on pace to account for future demands of urologic care. This impending urologic shortage sits on a backdrop of multiple other workforce issues. In this review, we take an in-depth look at several pressing issues facing the urologic workforce, including the impending urology shortage, gender and diversity concerns, growing levels of burnout, and the effects of the coronavirus pandemic. In doing so, we highlight specific areas of clinical practice that may need to be addressed from a health care policy standpoint.

**An Updated Review on Physician Burnout in Urology**     173

Jennifer Nauheim and Amanda C. North

> Physician burnout is an issue having an impact on all of medicine but having a significant impact on the field of urology. Burnout begins in medical school and worsens in residency. Increased workload leads to increased burnout both in residency and in practice. Issues with work-life balance, electronic medical record usage, decreasing reimbursements, and increased Centers for Medicare & Medicaid Services burden all have an impact on physician satisfaction with their practices. Burnout should be acknowledged, and measures for prevention should be taken by hospitals and residency programs to decrease and prevent physician burnout.

**Development of Physician Leaders**     179

Laura Crocitto, Deepak A. Kapoor, and Kevin R. Loughlin

> The complexity of health care today along with the drive towards value-based care are strong forces in support of growing and expanding the physician leadership workforce. Physician led organizations are associated with improved physician engagement, quality of care and cost efficiency. Physicians would benefit from more formal leadership training which incorporates a structed leadership curriculum, mentorship and on the job progressive leadership experience. Special attention must be placed on increasing the diversity of our physician leaders. There are many important characteristics to look for in our physician leaders including emotional intelligence, integrity, visioning, humility, persuasion and the ability to listen.

### Women in Urology                                                                    187

Mara R. Holton and Kari Bailey

The presence of women in genitourinary (GU) specialty training and practice has lagged significantly behind other fields. Current challenges include maternity leave, sexual harassment, and pay disparities. Despite these obstacles, the prevalence of women in GU specialty training has risen rapidly. One consequence of retiring male providers and higher numbers of female graduates will be a notable demographic shift in the percentage of GU care provided by these younger women. It will be essential to anticipate and acknowledge the unique concerns of this workforce, particularly in light of the concomitant aging of the US population and the associated increase in demand for GU care.

### Understanding the Millennial Physician                                             195

Jake Quarles and Jason Hafron

The millennial generation has become the largest generation thus far and continues to grow, as it makes up a substantial part of the workforce. Often misunderstood, those identifying as millennials offer skills, traits, and characteristics that previous generations have been unable to provide. Learning to understand these millennials and all they have to offer serves key to a successful training program or practice. A millennial's understanding of technology, grasp of patient-provider relationships, and desire to work hard contribute to their success as urologists.

### The Role of Advanced Practice Providers in Urology                                 203

Deepak A. Kapoor

The nation's undersupply of urology services disproportionately affects Medicare beneficiaries compared to the general population. Advanced Practice Providers (APPs), most commonly nurse practitioners and physician assistants may be a vehicle to meet this need. The increased use of APPs in urology is hampered by physician discomfort with delegating responsibility to APPs. This discomfort may be compounded by complexities with billing issues and interstate variation in scope of practice regulations. To expand access to urological services while simultaneously ensuring service quality, it is imperative that urologists engage with APPs individually and as a specialty.

### Telemedicine in Urology: The Socioeconomic Impact                                   215

Eric Kirshenbaum, Eugene Y. Rhee, Matthew Gettman, and Aaron Spitz

The emergence of the COVID-19 pandemic and subsequent public health emergency (PHE) have propelled telemedicine several years into the future. With the rapid adoption of this technology came socioeconomic inequities as minority communities disproportionately have yet to adopt telemedicine. Telemedicine offers solutions to patient access issues that have plagued urology, helping address physician shortages in rural areas and expanding the reach of urologists. The Centers for Medicare & Medicaid Services have adopted changes to expand coverage for telemedicine services. The expectation is that telemedicine will continue to be a mainstay in the health care system with gradual expansion in utilization.

**The Growth of Integrated Care Models in Urology**     223

Caitlin Shepherd, Michael Cookson, and Neal Shore

With heightened awareness of health care outcomes and efficiencies and reimbursement-based metrics, it is ever more important that urologists consider the effects of integrated care models on physicians/staff/clinics fulfillment and patient outcomes, and whether and how to optimally implement these models within their unique practice settings. Despite growing evidence that integrating care improves outcomes, uncertainty persists regarding which approach is most efficient and achievable in terms of specialty considerations and financial resources. In this article, we discuss strategies for integrating urologic care and its impact on current and future health care delivery.

**Private Equity and Urology: An Emerging Model for Independent Practice**     233

Gary M. Kirsh and Deepak A. Kapoor

Independent urology practices are under increasing competitive pressure in a changing marketplace. By providing access to capital and business management expertise, private equity can help practices consolidate and scale to unlock new growth opportunities, navigate an increasingly complex regulatory environment, and institute best practice across a network, while retaining physician ownership and an opportunity for equity appreciation. This article examines the role of private equity in urology and the potential benefits of private equity investment. It also looks at what firms look for in investment partners, how to prepare for private equity investment, and how private equity investments are structured.

**Clinical Research 2021**     245

Evan R. Goldfischer

Clinical research is of great benefit to patients and rewarding to clinicians. Clinical research in the United States is highly regulated. There are significant penalties for violating protocols. Clinical research requires a good infrastructure in each practice.

**Health Policy and Advocacy**     251

Thomas H. Rechtschaffen and Deepak A. Kapoor

Awareness of the activities of federal and state legislative and regulatory activities is vital for physicians to avoid having their services misvalued and to protect patients' access to care. Professional organizations are encouraging physicians to develop political leadership and advocacy skills to protect patient care, research, and access to technology. The political polarization of the country and the public health emergency have had an impact on the ability and willingness of some to engage in policy discussions. This article reviews mechanisms by which urologists can engage in health policy and political activity and avenues to expand the number of urologists involved.

**Current and Future Status of Merit-Based Incentive Payment Systems**     259

Kathleen L. Latino and Deepak A. Kapoor

The Quality Payment Program was established by the Medicare Access and CHIP Reauthorization Act (MACRA) legislation in response to repeated efforts to create a permanent so-called doc fix in response to the failures of the sustainable growth formula. This article examines the history leading up to MACRA, the current pathways associated with the Quality Payment Program, and future expectation both from the Centers for Medicare and Medicaid Services, stakeholders, and patients.

**Finance 101 for Physicians**                                                                 **269**

Christopher G. Stappas

Although physicians enjoy extensive educational backgrounds, financial planning typically is not a significant component of the curricula they have completed. As a result, many physicians could benefit from greater financial acumen, and their preparation for retirement might be lacking in light of their relatively high-income levels. This article by a private wealth advisor with 29 years of industry experience provides physicians with the basic building blocks to understand and manage their finances. It focuses on 3 pillars of financial planning: (1) protecting themselves, their families, and their assets; (2) reducing their taxes; and (3) growing their wealth.

# UROLOGIC CLINICS OF NORTH AMERICA

**FORTHCOMING ISSUES**

*August 2021*
**Prostate Cancer Genetics: Changing the Paradigm of Care**
Leonard G. Gomella and Veda Giri, *Editors*

*November 2021*
**Sexual Dysfunction: A New Era**
Alan W. Shindel and Tom F. Lue, *Editors*

*February 2022*
**Minimally Invasive Urology: Past, Present, and Future**
John Denstedt, *Editor*

**RECENT ISSUES**

*February 2021*
**Robotic Urology: The Next Frontier**
Jim C. Hu and Jonathan E. Shoag, *Editors*

*November 2020*
**Cancer Immunotherapy in Urology**
Sujit S. Nair and Ashutosh K. Tewari, *Editors*

*August 2020*
**Advanced and Metastatic Renal Cell Carcinoma**
William C. Huang and Ezequiel Becher, *Editors*

SERIES OF RELATED INTEREST
*Surgical Clinics of North America*
**https://www.surgical.theclinics.com/**

# UROLOGIC CLINICS OF NORTH AMERICA

## FORTHCOMING ISSUES

**August 2021**
Prostate Cancer Genetics: Changing the Paradigm of Care
Leonard G. Gomella and Veda Giri, Editors

**November 2021**
Sexual Dysfunction: A New Era
Alan W. Shindel and Tom F. Lue, Editors

**February 2022**
Minimally Invasive Urology: Past, Present, and Future
John Denstedt, Editor

## RECENT ISSUES

**February 2021**
Robotic Urology: The Next Frontier
Jim C. Hu and Jonathan E. Shoag, Editors

**November 2020**
Cancer Immunotherapy in Urology
Sujit S. Nair and Ashutosh K. Tewari, Editors

**August 2020**
Advanced and Metastatic Renal Cell Carcinoma
William C. Huang and Ezequiel Becher, Editors

SERIES OF RELATED INTEREST
Surgical Clinics of North America
https://www.surgical.theclinics.com/

# Foreword

# Between the Forty-Yard Lines: Health Care Reform and its Impact on the Changing Landscape of Urologic Practice

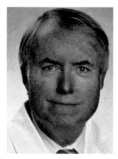

Kevin R. Loughlin, MD, MBA
*Consulting Editor*

Late last year, I had the opportunity to attend a Zoom interview of David Gergen. He has served in the administrations of both political parties and has been a keen observer of how things get done within the Beltway throughout his distinguished career. He is, in my opinion, a man of uncommon wisdom. During the interview, he shared that he thought that in Washington, DC most things get accomplished "between the forty-yard lines." I think it is an apt metaphor for the current political environment regarding health care reform, which is the underpinning for the changing landscape of urologic practice.

As we enter this year with a new president and a new congress, one of their major tasks will be health care reform. For the last several decades, this issue has dominated medical practice, and its lack of resolution has perpetuated an uncertainty that has permeated every aspect of our profession.

Virtually every topic that Dr Kapoor has selected for inclusion in this issue of *Urologic Clinics* on physician burnout: clinical research, workforce exigencies, physician leadership, the expanding role of advanced practice providers, and the growth of integrated care models, just to name a few, is a response to the economic exigencies that are the consequences of our unsettled and inefficient health care delivery.

Dr Kapoor, long a thought leader in urologic clinical practice, has created this issue that will serve as an ecphoneme for the challenges facing urologic practice now as well as provide insights into where we are headed in the future with possible solutions. The confluence of urologist burnout, workforce issues, the aging of the population, the incorporation of physician extenders, scribes, and telemedicine is changing urologic practice in profound, immutable ways.

As the new executive and legislative branches assume power, it is incumbent upon urologists to remain informed and engaged. The options for health care reform are fairly clear. There are those who are enthusiastic for some kind of single-payer health care, whether it is called Medicare for All or Universal Health Care, whereas others call for an expansion of Obamacare. Few want to maintain status quo.

A thorough evaluation of all our health care options is beyond the scope of this article, but I think certain premises seem obvious. Most people agree that access to health care is an essential component for a modern society. A reasonable underpinning for any future health care system would appear to be (1) transparency of costs, (2) competition, (3) access to care, (4) choice of provider and health care facility, and (5) protection of those with preexisting conditions.

Urol Clin N Am 48 (2021) xi–xiii
https://doi.org/10.1016/j.ucl.2021.02.003

urologic.theclinics.com

Former presidential candidate and Louisiana governor, Bobby Jindal, has opined that, "President Biden will be unable to pass a 'public option,' and Republicans will be unable to repeal the Affordable Care Act."[1] Is this a prediction of continued legislative gridlock?

However, it would appear that choices in the future likely will be permutations of Medicare for All versus an expansion of Obamacare. It is important to recognize that universal health care and single-payer health care are not synonymous.

## CURRENT SINGLE-PAYER TRIAL BALLOONS

Recent single-payer health care proposals, at a state level, have not met with success. In November 2016, Amendment 69, ColoradoCare, proposed a single-payer, government-run system and was soundly defeated by an almost 4-to-1 margin.[2]) Despite outspending its opponents by an almost 5-to-1 margin, ColoradoCare gained very little voter traction. Post–election analysis showed that a major reason for the lack of voter traction was cost and that Colorado voters understood that a $25 billion tax increase to provide "free" health care was a fantasy.

In Vermont, Green Mountain Health (H.202) would have required an 11% increased payroll tax and was abandoned.[3] In California, S.B. 562, Healthy California, was estimated to have a cost ranging from $331 to $400 billion and was not pursued.[4]

The term "Medicare for All" has often been used imprecisely by the media and some politicians. There really are 2 models for Medicare for All: the pure model and the hybrid model[5] The pure model of Medicare for All aims to establish a national insurance program operated by the federal government and explicitly prohibits private insurance for services covered by the publicly funded government plan. The hybrid model allows private insurance plans that adhere to federal regulations, including those sponsored by employers, to operate alongside and within a government-run Medicare program.[5] It is also important to realize that no Medicare for All plan would actually cover all Americans. The pure model proposed by Senator Sanders provides that both the Veterans Health Administration and the Indian Health Service would remain intact.[5]

## LESSONS FROM THE CANADIAN EXPERIENCE

First, it should be acknowledged that the population of Canada is 37 million, whereas the population of California is 39 million and the United States is 329 million.[6] The origins of Canadian universal care began in Saskatchewan in 1947. This evolved into 13 provincial and territorial plans financed by per-capita block grants from the federal government.

These plans culminated in the Canadian Health Act of 1984, which initially outlawed private insurance and allowed no additional charges by physicians.[7] It should be recognized that the legislation was 14 pages compared with 900 pages for Obamacare, and the Canadian legislation was passed by a vote of 177 to 2.

Although the Canadian plan incorporates many attractive features, wait times have always been problematic even with their smaller and less urban population. Pipes[8] reports that the median time for a patient to be seen by a specialist after a general practitioner referral was 21.2 weeks, more than double the wait time of 25 years ago. The government has tacitly approved of patients paying private clinics out of their own pockets, and private clinics perform more than 60,000 operations a year, saving the public treasury $240 million.[8]

## THE LOSS OF PRIVATE HEALTH INSURANCE FALL OUT

A single-payer system has some undeniable advantages. Physicians spend an average of 142 hours annually interacting with health plans at a cost to practices of $68,274 per physician.[9] There are 9 times more clerical workers in health care than physicians and 2 times as many workers as nurses.[10] When compared with Canada and 6 European nations, US hospital administrative costs are by far the highest.[10]

In addition, private health insurance employs about 500,000 people, and these people would have to be retrained and, in many cases relocated, if private insurance was abandoned.[11] Medicare and Medicaid pay hospitals about 87% to 90% of their actual costs, and hospitals shift costs to private insurers, which tend to pay 140% of costs.[11] Abelson and Sanger-Katz[12] concluded, "The real savings of Medicare for All would come from paying doctors and hospitals less than their cost of treating patients." Many of those private health insurance companies are major components of IRAs and stock investments for millions of Americans. Elizabeth Rosenthal[13] has further cautioned that under a single-payer system, most hospitals and specialists would lose money. She suggests that 5000 community hospitals would lose more than $151 billion.

President Biden advocates a preservation of the essentials of Obamacare with an expansion of it by including a public option that would serve as an alternative for Americans without insurance and those with employer-sponsored or individually purchased by some consumers to receive their health insurance. As is often said, the devil is in the details; the costs of this option remain uncertain as well as whether it would actually achieve universal coverage.

## THE PATH FORWARD

The purpose of this foreword is not to present a précis of health care options. Rather, it is to present, in broad brush strokes, the issues that will need to be considered in any health reform proposal. The Senate is divided 50/50 by party, and the country is divided to a degree as only rarely seen in our history. The US Census Bureau[14] reports that in 2018, 8.5% of Americans or 27.5 million Americans did not have health insurance at any point during the year. The most important message is to heed the wisdom of David Gergen. Our elected officials, on both sides of the aisle, have failed us in the past. As we enter the terms of a new president and a new congress, 1 thing appears certain: the status quo is untenable. Meaningful health care reform is long overdue. Going forward, our legislative leaders need to incorporate the views of physicians, far more than previously, as to practical solutions to the health care crisis. They need to listen to Gergen, that compromise and consensus are fundamental to all successful legislation. Yes, important yardage can be gained between the forty-yard lines, and if you work it right, you may even score a touchdown.

Kevin R. Loughlin, MD, MBA
Vascular Biology Research Program at
Boston Children's Hospital
300 Longwood Avenue
Boston, MA 02115, USA

*E-mail address:*
kloughlin@partners.org

## REFERENCES

1. Jindal B. Can GOP find its way on health care? Wall Street Journal. December 3, 2020; section A;3.
2. Ray K. ColoradoCare suffered a whopping defeat. Here's why. Available at: https://www.coloradoindependent.com/2016/11/08/coloradocare-amendment-69/. Accessed October 10, 2020.
3. Vermont health care reform. Available at: https://en.wikipedia.org/wiki/Vermont_health_care_reform. Accessed October 10, 2020.
4. S.B. 562 The Healthy California Act (2017-2018). Available at: https://leginfo.legislative.ca.gov/faces/billNavClient.xhtml?bill_id=20172018SB562. Accessed October 10, 2020.
5. Oberlander J. Navigating the shifting terrain of U.S. Health Care Reform—Medicare For All, single payer, and the public option. Milbank Q 2019;1–15.
6. Wikipedia. List of countries by population. Available at: https://en.wikipedia.org/wiki/List_of_countries_by_population_(United Nations. Accessed October 11, 2020.
7. Naylor CD. Canada as single-payer exemplar for universal health care in the United States: a borderline option. JAMA 2018;319(1):17–8.
8. Pipes SC. Single-payer health care isn't worth waiting for. Wall Street Journal. January 22, 2018.
9. Casalino LP. What does it cost physician practices to interact with health insurance plans? Health Aff 2009;28(4):w533–43.
10. Himmelstein DU, et al. A comparison of hospital administrative costs in eight nations: U.S. costs exceed all others by far. Health Aff 2014;33(9):1586–94.
11. Medicare for all bailout. Wall Street Journal. Editorial. August 15, 2019.
12. Abelson R, Sanger-Katz M. Idea would end private insurance, then what? New York Times. March 20, 2019.
13. Rosenthal E. The costs of reform. New York Times. May 20, 2019.
14. Berchick ER, Barnett JC, Upton RD. Health care coverage in the United States: 2018. November 8, 2019. Report number P60-267(RV). United States Census Bureau.

# Preface

# Embracing Change in Urologic Practice: Both Without and Within

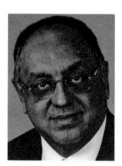

Deepak A. Kapoor, MD
*Editor*

This is the only the second time that this prestigious publication has devoted an entire issue to the socioeconomics of health care. Given the upheaval associated with the global Public Health Emergency and the current political uncertainty in the country, the timing of the *Urologic Clinics* for such a review couldn't be more appropriate. The protective bubble that has sheltered physicians from the harsh economic realities other professions face has burst—not only have we seen our livelihoods threatened but also our very lives as front-line workers are at risk as we minister to our patients. In this environment, nascent issues of access, diversity, and leadership have been brought into sharp focus. It was a great honor to have been asked by Dr. Loughlin to serve as guest editor to review these matters in this august journal. I've had the distinct privilege of working with all the authors who have contributed to this issue in various capacities over the last several years, each of whom is an authority on their respective topic—their individual and collective contributions to the field are too numerous to list, and I am sure that you will find their insights invaluable.

This issue of the *Urologic Clinics* is loosely organized into sections generally focusing on workforce and enhancing access, novel practice structures and opportunities, advocacy, and finance. The first section starts with 2 studies of the present state of the urologic workforce, exploring not only the absolute need for urologic services but also the increased pressure on access to care that results from physician burnout. These are followed by 4 reviews of possible methods to enhance access to care, through coordinated efforts in development of physician leaders, enhancing the role of women in urology, nurturing the next generation of urologic physicians, and the opportunities and challenges in expanding the use of advanced practice providers. The last article in this section covers the history and future of telemedicine, the role of which was catapulted into prominence over this last year.

The next section focuses on opportunities for urologists outside of traditional practice structures. This starts with the evolution of integrated care models, which now account for over a third of the nation's urologic services. This is followed by a study exploring the upsurge of private equity transactions in health care—over $80 billion worth of deals closed in the health care space in the year prior to the COVID-19 crisis. Next is an overview of operationalizing research programs into clinical practice, an opportunity that most urologists do not avail themselves to.

The subsequent 2 articles start with a primer on engagement in advocacy, exploring different approaches taken by different urologic associations, mechanisms by which urologists can engage in the process, and case studies that illustrate the evolution of urologic advocacy—the adage "if you're not at the table, you'll be on the menu"

Urol Clin N Am 48 (2021) xv–xvi
https://doi.org/10.1016/j.ucl.2021.02.002
0094-0143/21/© 2021 Published by Elsevier Inc.

has never been truer. We move to an overview of the status of the Merit-based Incentive Payment System and current regulations to help readers comply with provisions of the Medicare Access and CHIP Reauthorization Act of 2012. Given the economic uncertainties faced by physicians, it seemed appropriate to finish this issue with an overview of basic financial planning, a subject that is sorely lacking in medical education.

While we are first and foremost scientists and practitioners of an ancient art, as the principal caregivers of the genitourinary tract, we must serve as advocates for both our patients and those that will follow in our profession. As such, we must ensure continued access to our services while securing professional satisfaction and economic security for current and future practitioners. To do so, we must remain vigilant to changes in the practice climate, educate ourselves on issues affecting our specialty and our patients, and, most importantly, embrace our role as agents of change for the betterment of our patients and profession.

Deepak A. Kapoor, MD
Integrated Medical Professionals
Solaris Health Holdings, LLC
The Icahn School of Medicine at
Mount Sinai
340 Broadhollow Road
Farmingdale, NY 11735, USA

*E-mail address:*
dkapoor@imppllc.com

# Workforce Issues in Urology

Ryan Dornbier, MD*, Christopher M. Gonzalez, MD, MBA

## KEYWORDS

• Workforce • Burnout • COVID-19 • Urology shortage • Diversity • Equality

## KEY POINTS

- There will be a substantial shortage of urologists in the near future affecting rural communities more so than urban areas.
- The urologic workforce lacks in diversity and needs to make additional efforts to recruit and maintain women and underrepresented minorities.
- Burnout is an ever-growing issue among urologists, which may affect productivity and desire to continue in the workforce.
- As the we begin to recover from the COVID-19 pandemic, the urologic workforce needs to be adaptable and innovative in its response.

## INTRODUCTION

The American Urologic Association (AUA) publishes a yearly report entitled "The State of the Urology Workforce and Practice in the United States." The information, compiled from the AUA Annual Census, offers insight into urologic workforce trends through an ever-broadening scope of topics including demographics, geographic distribution, compensation, practice characteristics, and financial profiles. The most recent iteration of this report, stemming from the 2019 AUA Annual Census, was published in April 2020.[1] Through this lens, a variety of urologic workforce issues have been brought into focus; some building for many years, and others have become increasingly apparent.

As of 2019, there were 13,044 practicing urologists of whom 11,167 (85.6%) were active urologists working more than 25 hours per week. The number of practicing urologists has gradually increased since 2014 (**Fig. 1**).[1–6] However, these numbers offer a misleading perspective. The active urologist-to-population ratio has not increased at the level needed to care for the growing population (see **Fig. 1**, red line). Therefore, there is a significant concern for an impending urologist shortage, in

line with the impending global shortage of physicians.[7] This shortage exists on the backdrop of an existing geographic maldistribution of urologists that will affect rural communities more severely than urban locations.[8,9]

In addition to the geographic imbalance and relative decline of actively practicing urologists to match the growing population, there are significant concerns regarding the diversity of the urologic workforce. As of 2019, female providers make up only 9.9% of the workforce.[1] Although this percentage has been steadily increasing over the past several years, it still represents a significant shortcoming of women urologists. Furthermore, the racial makeup of the urologic workforce is substantially disproportionate to the US population.[1] Outside of absolute shortages and diversity concerns, the urologic workforce is dealing with the fallout of the coronavirus pandemic in 2020. For many, this has resulted in postponement of elective surgeries to divert resources to the care of patients with Coronavirus Disease 2019 (COVID-19). Unfortunately, this has led to a significant decline in clinical activity in both the surgical and clinic settings for many. As of this writing, the initial consequences appear to be a backlog of elective

Department of Urology, Stritch School of Medicine, Loyola University Medical Center, 2160 S. First Ave., Maywood, IL 60153, USA
* Corresponding author.
*E-mail address:* ryan.dornbier@lumc.edu

Urol Clin N Am 48 (2021) 161–171
https://doi.org/10.1016/j.ucl.2021.01.001
0094-0143/21/© 2021 Elsevier Inc. All rights reserved.

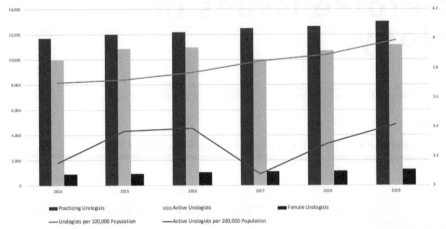

**Fig. 1.** Practicing, active, and female urologists in the United States with urologist-to-population ratio measured in urologists per 100,000 population. (*Data from* the AUA State of the Urology Workforce and Practice in the United States from 2014-2019.)

procedures, decreased urologic productivity, and repurposing of urologists to care for patients with COVID-19.[10] The long-term consequences of the pandemic have yet to be realized; however, as the financial toll of the pandemic reveals itself, so too will the impact on the urologic workforce.

The urologic community faces an ever-changing patient and societal environment. It is incumbent on us to continually evaluate our community and adapt to these needs. In this review, we take an in-depth look at several pressing issues facing the urologic workforce, including the impending urology shortage, gender and diversity concerns, growing levels of burnout, and the effects of the coronavirus pandemic. In doing so, we highlight specific areas of clinical practice that may need to be addressed from a health care policy standpoint.

## UROLOGY SHORTAGE

The demand for urologic care is relatively predictable. The American population is growing and aging. The US Census Bureau estimates that nearly 56.1 million Americans are older than 65, representing 17% of the population. This percentage is projected to increase to 21% by 2030, and 23% by 2060.[11] Moreover, urology is largely a specialty providing care to older adults. The Centers for Disease Control and Prevention estimated that in 2016 there were 23 million office visits for urologic care, 52.6% were for individuals 65 or older.[12,13] Naturally, it follows that with a growing and aging population, the demand for urologic care will increase.

The supply of urologic care is less predictable and contingent on 2 factors. First, the overall supply of urologists, which is subject to the same economic forces that influence other labor markets. This includes the current supply of urologists, minus those leaving the workforce, plus those

entering the workforce (**Fig. 2**). There are multiple factors that influence these metrics, with urologist retirement patterns and residency training positions driving a large degree of the equation. Second, urologic care supply is influenced by the individual productivity in terms of the number of patients seen and hours worked. Metrics, such as burn out, greater interest in work-life balance, and aging, may influence overall quantity of work, further limiting urologic care supply.

The aging of the urologic workforce drives a substantial concern regarding the impending urology shortage. As of the 2019 AUA Census, 52% of urologists are older than 55, making urology the second oldest specialty after cardiothoracic surgery.[1] Furthermore, roughly 27% of practicing urologists plan to retire within the next 5 years.[14] Retirement, at present, is a personal choice for the individual surgeon, although as a person ages, there is a natural decline in cognitive and physical function. Policy regarding the optimal age of retirement is not widespread; however, with age comes decreased clinical production. Older urologists see fewer patients on a weekly basis.[15,16] In addition, some older urologists may prefer to decrease operative volume, while maintaining their clinic schedule. At present, 33.1% of urologists who do not perform inpatient surgery cite age/retirement as a reason.[1] Therefore, even if older urologists elect to forego retirement, their practice patterns will likely exhibit a decline in volume.[17] This volume reduction adds to the shortage in urologic care.

Given current trends, scarcity of urologists will be profound in the near future. The US Department of Health and Human Services predicts a shortage of 3630 urologists by 2025.[18] In a similar report from the *Annals of Surgery*, the field will fall 3880 full-time equivalents (FTE) short, or 32% fewer than the projected need.[19] This will place the

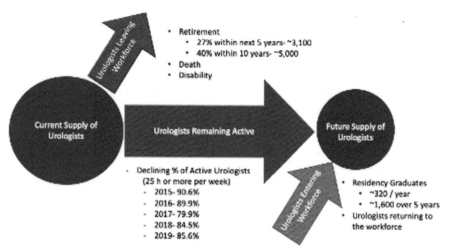

**Fig. 2.** Factors influencing the supply of urologists in the United States.

urologist-to-population ratio at 2.24 per 100,000 (compared with 3.99/100,000 in 2019), well below a sustainable level and inconsistent with future need.[20] Needless to say, a crisis exists for the future of access to care, with uncertain implications on quality and outcomes, for benign and life-threatening urologic conditions.

With growing demand relatively certain, addressing the supply of the urologic workforce becomes imperative. However, bolstering the supply of urologists is fraught with limitations, both logistically and financially. First, it is unrealistic, to expect and rely on older urologists to continue to prolong their careers. It seems the simplest solution would be to ensure that the retiring urologist is replaced by a newly and adequately trained graduating resident. Over the past 8 match cycles, the AUA reports an average of 308 matched residents each year, ranging from 279 to 353.[21] To alleviate the projected 2030 FTE shortage over the next 10 years (388 additional graduates per year), urology programs would have to more than double present class capacity, an unrealistic addition of approximately 2.5 residents per program per year. This is both educationally and financially unachievable. In 1997, Congress passed the Balanced Budget Act capping the number of residency spots funded by the federal government. Since that time, Medicare, Medicaid, and the Department of Veterans Affairs has funded 170 urology residency positions each year.[22] The remaining funds have come from clinical revenue, hospital funds, medical schools, philanthropy, or departments themselves.[22,23] Estimates place the cost of training additional residents to meet future need at more than $3 billion, a price not easily absorbed without government assistance.[19] There is some optimism that a portion of this financial burden may be alleviated by the Resident Physician Shortage Reduction Act of 2019, a bill that has received bipartisan support for the addition of 15,000 residency positions, half of which will be used for shortage specialty residency programs.[24] However, without substantial funding and increased faculty to support educational quality, alternative solutions are necessary to ease the urology shortage.

With the impractical idea of increasing graduating residents in the short term, one area of interest is the increased utilization of advanced practice providers (APPs), physician assistants or nurse practitioners, to ease the urology workforce shortage. Over the past 20 years, APPs have seen a marked increase in number, as well as an increase in responsibility.[25] This includes performing office-based and minor local procedures and utilization as surgical assistants.[26,27] This expansion of APP utilization has shown to improve patient access and decrease new patient wait times[28]; however, it is often at the expense of formalized training.[29,30] APPs have limitations on the scope of their abilities, as most work in an ambulatory setting and are not trained to perform more complex inpatient care.[31] The utilization of APPs is discussed more extensively in other articles in this issue; nonetheless, APPs are critical members of the team-based approach to urologic care, which is necessary to meet increasing patient demand, and should be under the direct supervision of a board-certified urologist.

### Urology Shortage in Rural America

Nowhere is the impending urology shortage more dire than in nonmetropolitan areas; 19.2% of the US population lives in rural areas, whereas only 10.4% of urologists work in nonmetropolitan areas, with 0.4% classifying their practice as rural.[1] This leaves a substantial shortage in many areas of the country. In total, 62.4% of American counties have zero practicing urologists. In addition, urologists working in nonmetropolitan areas are older and closer to retirement than their urban counterparts.[1,22,32] Nearly a third of rural urologists work in a solo practice, a concerning figure in that their eventual retirement will leave a significant void in their community.[32]

Replacing the rural urologist seems a difficult endeavor. Urology residents are not eager to enter practice in rural settings. In the AUA 2019 Urologists in Training Census Book, only 3.1% of residents were considering rural practice.[33] Recruitment obstacles to rural urology are likely similar to those for other surgical specialties, including increasingly specialized training, increased workload, higher call burden, shifting generational desires, more expensive malpractice coverage, and decreased reimbursements.[34–37] With limited providers, there are growing concerns that the urban-rural divide will only deepen, leading to undertreatment and worse outcomes.[38–40]

Solutions to the rural urology crisis will need to be multimodal. Overall, strategies will need to be wide in scope and advanced to appropriately mitigate the impending shortage with involvement of recruiting, outreach, and alternative care efforts (**Fig. 3**). Telemedicine appears to be an opportunity for easy remote outreach, while allowing for shorter travel distances and relatively high patient satisfaction.[41] Telemedicine offers low cost and efficient care delivery with relatively few pitfalls. Internet access, technical literacy, Health Insurance Portability and Accountability Act (HIPAA) compliance, and insurance coverage issues have previously limited telemedicine utilization.[42] However, with the rapid relaxation of regulatory and reimbursement barriers caused by the COVID-19 pandemic, urologists may have an opportunity to implement telemedicine into routine practice and allow for greater rural outreach.[43]

APPs have been used in rural settings for primary care and emergency department care.[44,45] This solution has the same pitfalls as previously discussed when addressing the national urologist shortage. Moreover, the idea of APPs practicing in a rural setting is complicated by variability in scope of practice legislation from state to state. As mentioned previously, APPs in urology should work in a formally defined alliance with a urologist serving in a supervisory role[46]; however, states with restrictive regulations may limit an APP's ability to practice effectively in rural settings without any urology presence. For APPs to be effectively used in rural locations, states would need to allow for less restrictive practice regulations; however, it is paramount that this is done in a coordinated and collaborative agreement with a supervising urologist.[25] In this way, APPs in the rural setting could

allow for triaged care and performance of some office-based procedures.

Unfortunately, long-term, sustainable solutions must rely on the recruitment of fully trained urologists to rural and underserved settings. Nationally subsidized loan forgiveness, increased reimbursement, and implementation of rural rotations in residency may incentivize graduating residents to practice in rural locations. Other strategies rely on focused recruitment efforts by targeting medical students from rural communities for urology residency spots.[33] A key determinant for entering rural practice is often growing up in a rural setting; thus, seeking trainees from these locations may lead to increased interest.[34] Another targeted recruitment option involves recruitment of International Medical Graduates (IMGs) for future work in rural locations. Most IMGs in the United States enter residency on a J-1 visa nonimmigrant exchange program. At the conclusion of training, IMGs must return to their home country for a 2-year period before applying for a new visa in the United States. Alternatively, the IMG can seek a J-1 visa waiver by working for the 2-year period in a medically underserved area. This often constitutes a rural location. Therefore, if urology residencies increase the number of IMGs, there may be incentive for proceeding to practice in rural locations.[20,47] However, the number of IMGs in the urologic workforce and residency training programs has declined over the past 25 years.[20,47] Moreover, retention of IMGs in rural locations may be difficult due to a lack of integration within certain communities.[48]

A more aggressive approach to the rural urology shortage would be the establishment of rural residency programs or rural urology tracks. This would be a more expansive effort than rural urology rotations in residency, but instead placing resident acceptance into a residency spot contingent on future practice in a rural setting. This has been attempted in the general surgery residency match with moderate success.[49,50] This format may attract medical students interested in rural urology, especially those from rural settings. There are a multitude of different approaches to starting and funding such residency tracks; however, if the rural shortage becomes more dire, aggressive recruitment strategies may be necessary.

## DIVERSITY AND GENDER WORKFORCE ISSUES
### Diversity in Urology

The urologic workforce does not reflect the ethnic makeup of the United States. The racial makeup of the urologic community is 84.7% white, 11.7% Asian, 2.0% Black, and 1.6% other races. In a

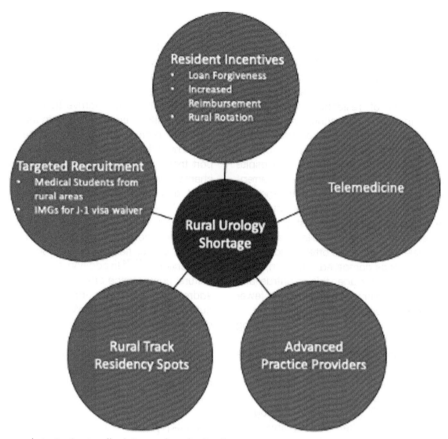

**Fig. 3.** Proposed strategies to alleviate rural urologist shortage.

separate categorization of ethnicity, only 3.9% of respondents identified as Hispanic.[1] Therefore, Black and Hispanic individuals make up just 5.9% of the urologic workforce (this percentage may be lower, as the categorizations are not mutually exclusive). This national trend is replicated in every AUA section.[51] This is unlikely to change in the near term; according to the AUA resident census, 3.1% and 5.7% of current residents report being Black or Hispanic, respectively.[33] Urology significantly lags behind other surgical specialties and medical fields in the proportion of minority members and trainees.[52]

This lack of diversity in urology and among urologic trainees stems from a multitude of unique challenges facing minorities throughout the medical training process. Most residency programs lack a curriculum or mentorship programs to address diversity issues.[53] Minorities have reported encounters with implicit and explicit bias by faculty, patients, and staff that leads to burnout and stressful training environments.[54] These racial biases in health care extend far beyond the training period[55]; as such, minority populations experience a continuation of adverse and challenging work environments throughout their career. This suggests that minority populations may learn and work in a less supportive atmosphere and are subjected to racial harassment and discrimination, sometimes routinely.[56]

## Women in Urology

For many years, urology has been a male-dominated specialty, and currently ranks last in terms of percentage of female physicians when compared with other specialties.[57] There has been a gradual increase in the number of female urologists over the past 10 years (see **Fig. 1**), with current data showing 9.9% of the workforce is female. Optimism exists that this number will continue to grow. Of urologists younger than 45 years, 22.2% are female.[1] Even more encouraging, 29.4% of urology residents are female.[33] Estimates project that by 2035, approximately 25% of the urologic workforce will be made up of female providers,[9] with consistent growth over the next 4 decades.[58] Despite these marginal improvements, urology still has a difficult time recruiting female medical students and lags behind almost all surgical subspecialties in percentage of female residents.[54,59]

As much as the number of women entering the field is increasing, female urologists face an ever-growing set of challenges and gender differences. Foremost is the discrepancy in compensation; female urologists make approximately $80,000 less per year than their male counterparts.[60] Female residents also anticipate a lower annual compensation on completion of residency, with 67.6% expecting less than $350,000 annually compared with 58.6% of male residents.[33] More female urologists are fellowship trained and a higher proportion work primarily in an academic setting.[1,61,62] Despite this academic achievement, women are underrepresented in academic leadership roles and are less likely to achieve academic promotion.[63,64] The female urologist is often typecast into caring for female patients and female urologic issues.[65] Moreover, female urologists are often criticized for working fewer hours as compared with men; however, when controlling for age, this is untrue and likely reflective of younger urologists working fewer hours than their older counterparts.[61]

In the face of these challenges, women pursuing urology often make considerable sacrifice. Compared with the general population, female urologists give birth later, have more pregnancy complications, greater infertility issues, and are more likely to require assisted reproductive technologies to conceive.[66] Many female urologists delay motherhood until after training and have fewer children.[67] This often relates to a lack of satisfactory maternity leave policies and a lack of work-related modifications near term.[67] These sacrifices often stem from finding an appropriate balance between professional and home life. In an effort to attract more women to the field, it becomes important to minimize, if not eliminate, these challenges and sacrifices.

### Strategies to Improve Diversity and Gender in Urology

Increased diversity in the urologic workforce fosters a community of inclusion that benefits patient care and the workforce itself. By expanding the racial, ethnic, and gender profile of our community, we offer a more well-rounded and comprehensive training. This allows for more culturally sensitive care, improved outcomes for underserved populations, and more equitable solutions to a myriad of health care problems.[68–70] In this sense, it is important to recruit men and women from diverse cultural and ethnic backgrounds to careers in urology.

Efforts to cultivate a diverse workforce are not without strategy. This includes the recruitment and support of minorities and women throughout medical school, training, and practice to ensure that diversity is maintained.[54] This is often influenced by early exposure to urology through focused recruitment of minorities and women during the early years of medical school.[71] Other specialties have seen an increase in residency applications through mentorship programs and directed clerkships.[72] In addition, promoting a multicultural and supportive training environment through cultural education will, in itself, help to recruit a more multicultural and diverse workforce.[73]

The retention of a diverse workforce requires support throughout training and practice. This means championing national organizations for development and promotion of women and minorities, finding alternative methods for promotion that include mentorship and teaching endeavors, and developing concrete parental leave policies that support career flexibility for those that choose to have children.[60,74] In addition, this means promoting cultural competence among all practitioners[53] and addressing workplace biases and harassment quickly and effectively.[75] With increased efforts of diversity and inclusion, as previously discussed, the urology workforce will recruit, support, and retain a growing number of minority and female urologists. This will help develop a more culturally competent and balanced workforce for the care of an increasingly diverse and multicultural patient population.

## BURNOUT

Burnout is a condition characterized by the triad of emotional exhaustion, depersonalization, and decreased sense of accomplishment.[76] The causes of physician burnout often relate to dissatisfaction with work-life balance and job-related stressors, which include increased patient volume with shrinking reimbursement, longer hours with more time spent on clerical work, increased administrative demands, and lack of autonomy.[77,78] The effects of burnout include negative impact on quality of care, higher incidence of medical errors, reduced productivity, higher turnover, alcohol abuse, and, in severe cases, suicide.[79–81] Urologists report high rates of burnout. The 2016 AUA Census revealed a burnout rate of 38.8%.[4,76] According to Medscape's National Physician Burnout and Suicide Report of 2020, 54% of urologists report burnout, higher than any other specialty.[82] The implications of such high rates of burnout among the urology workforce are unknown. The speculation is that burnout will lead to increased urologist turnover through trainee dropout, decreased productivity, withdrawal from clinical work, or early retirement, all of which will add increased strain to an already diminished workforce.[78,83]

Amelioration of burnout requires identification of workplace stressors with attempts to ease pressures and improve coping mechanisms. Unfortunately, urologists in different practice settings and training levels experience burnout in different ways, such as studies that reveal that younger urologists in a private practice setting are more likely to experience burnout as compared with their older, academic colleagues.[78,84] For urologists as a whole, increasing work hours and quantity of work, almost universally, lead to increased levels of burnout, as longer time spent working allows for less time in self-care activities.[76,85] Moreover, increasing work hours with administrative or non–value-added tasks worsen burnout significantly.[76,86] Outside of adjustments to clinical duties and administrative tasks, it is important for urologists to routinely engage in self-care activities, such as exercising and interpersonal collaboration; this is associated with improved quality of life and has a positive impact on burnout.[76,84]

## EFFECTS OF THE CORONAVIRUS PANDEMIC

Most urologic workforce issues occur in an insidious manner, which requires long-term solutions or gradual adaptation. This could not be more different from the present COVID-19 pandemic. As of this writing, SARS-CoV-2 has infected nearly 25 million people and caused nearly 850,000 deaths worldwide, with 6 million cases and more than 180,000 deaths in the United States alone.[87] The resulting global health crisis has required rapid and unprecedented modifications to societal and medical norms in an effort to prevent viral transmission. This has resulted in a shortage of care for non-COVID medical issues and financial fallout.[88] Urologic services were variably impacted on a worldwide scale.[10] Largely this resulted in a reduction of outpatient clinic and surgical procedures to prevent unnecessary exposure and preserve a strained supply of personal protective equipment. Recommendations for triaging of urologic diagnoses for limitation of elective and nonemergent inpatient and outpatient procedures became necessary.[89–92] Meanwhile, many urologists in highly impacted regions were repurposed to care for patients with COVID-19.[10]

The impact to the urologic workforce in the United States was no less drastic. As of May 2020, approximately 2% of urologists had contracted the virus. In a survey conducted by the AUA, a strong majority of respondents reported a decrease in surgical volume and clinic volume (**Table 1**).[93] Almost two-thirds were operating at less than 10% of their pre-COVID surgical volume, whereas nearly 20% were not operating at all. Economically, many urologists reported reduced compensation or staff cuts to cope with the

financial fallout of the pandemic. In more severe circumstances, some urologists have been laid off or plan to retire because of the pandemic.[93] A small percentage of AUA members had transitioned to COVID-19 care,[93] whereas trainees were repurposed at approximately 26%. These numbers were higher in more highly affected areas.[94] Furthermore, many urologists shifted the way in which they provide care. Telemedicine has expanded exponentially during the pandemic, with many anticipating long-term and sustained usage of virtual visits.[95]

The emotional toll of the pandemic is also substantial. Most AUA members have experienced increased stress related to the pandemic. This largely reflects concern about COVID-19 exposure, the prospect of infection while working, or infecting others because of their work with significant mental health issues as a result of the pandemic.[93] Globally, nearly half of urologists felt fearful when going to work or felt inadequately trained to care for patients with COVID-19.[10]

The full impact of the pandemic, both on patient outcomes and economically, will not be fully realized for some time. Hospital systems and practices will likely feel the financial strain as they begin to return to pre-COVID levels of care. For many urologists, the concern has now shifted to the management of those patients who delayed care during the height of the pandemic to date. Some urologists report difficulty meeting the demand of backlogged procedures,[96] whereas others have expressed concern

| Table 1 Summary of results from the American Urologic Association "COVID-19 urology impact survey" | |
|---|---|
| **AUA Member Impact of COVID-19** | **Percentage** |
| Testing positive for COVID-19 | 2 |
| Reporting increased stress | 75 |
| Challenged by mental health concerns | 76 |
| Transitioned to care of patients with COVID-19 | 13 |
| *AUA member practice impact* | |
| Decreased surgical volume | 86 |
| Decreased clinical hours | 84 |
| Reduced compensation | 40 |
| Experiencing pay cut | 37 |
| Not receiving paycheck | 14 |
| Laid off | 4 |
| Plan to retire | 3 |
| Plan to close practice | 3 |

regarding delay in oncologic care leading to worse outcomes or more advanced disease at the time of presentation.[97] This will all fall over the backdrop of a system shocked by a loss of revenue from cancellation of elective procedures, functioning with reduced staff, loss of patient employment, and limited funds for capital expenditures.[98] In addition, fears of a "second wave" leads to further concern of shutdowns and reallocation of resources that could further shock the system. Overall, as the pandemic shifts from mitigation to recovery, it remains important for the urologic workforce to be adaptable and innovative in its response.

## SUMMARY

The urologic workforce faces many pressing concerns. The impending shortage of urologists, both overall and in rural areas, will cause significant strain over the course of the next several decades. This shortage exists on the backdrop of a workforce suffering from a significant lack of diversity that may further limit care to specific patient populations. As we recover from the COVID-19 pandemic, it will be important for urologists to confront these issues with active strategies for recruitment and inclusion to ensure the best quality of care for our patients.

## CLINICS CARE POINTS

- Due to the retirement of a large portion of older urologists over the next 5 years, there is a projected shortage of roughly 3600 urologists by 2025.
- The projected shortage of urologists will affect rural communities far more significantly, as urologists in rural areas tend to be older and closer to retirement than urologists practicing in metropolitan areas.
- Underlying the urologist shortage is a workforce that lacks representation of female and minority urologists.
- Challenges of future workforce development include the expansion of the racial, ethnic, and gender profile of the urologic community in an effort to care for an increasingly diverse and multicultural patient population.
- All of these concerns are present in a workforce experiencing a substantial degree of burnout and acutely affected by the emotional, economic, and health-related consequences of the COVID-19 pandemic.

## DISCLOSURE

The authors have nothing to disclose.

## REFERENCES

1. American Urological Association. The state of the urology workforce and practice in the United States 2019. Maryland: Linthicum; 2020.
2. American Urological Association. The state of the urology workforce and practice in the United States 2018. Maryland: Linthicum; 2019.
3. American Urological Association. The state of the urology workforce and practice in the United States 2017. Maryland: Linthicum; 2018.
4. American Urological Association. The state of the urology workforce and practice in the United States 2016. Maryland: Linthicum; 2017.
5. American Urological Association. The state of the urology workforce and practice in the United States 2015. Maryland: Linthicum; 2016.
6. American Urological Association. The state of the urology workforce and practice in the United States 2014. Maryland: Linthicum; 2015.
7. Crisp N, Chen L. Global supply of health professionals. N Engl J Med 2014;370:950–7.
8. Dall TM, Gallo PD, Chakrabarti R, et al. An aging population and growing disease burden will require a large and specialized health care workforce By 2025. Health Aff 2013;32:2013–20.
9. McKibben MJ, Kirby EW, Langston J, et al. Projecting the urology workforce over the next 20 years. Urology 2016;98:21–6.
10. Teoh JY-C, Ong WLK, Gonzalez-Padilla D, et al. A global survey on the impact of COVID-19 on urological services. Eur Urol 2020;78:265–75.
11. Vespa J, Medina L, Armstrong DM. Demographic turning points for the United States: population projections for 2020 to 2060. United States Census Bureau; 2020.
12. Anon. National Center for Health Statistics urology fact sheet from the National Ambulatory Medical Care Survey. Centers for Disease Control and Prevention. 2020. Available at: https://www.cdc.gov/nchs/data/namcs/factsheets/NAMCS_2015_16_Urology-508.pdf. Accessed June 17, 2020.
13. Rui POT. National Ambulatory Medical Care Survey: 2016 national summary tables. 2019. Available at: https://www.cdc.gov/nchs/data/ahcd/namcs_summary/2016_namcs_web_tables.pdf. Accessed June 17, 2020.
14. Gaither T, Awad M, Fang R, et al. MP37-11 The near future impact of retirement on the urologic workforce: results from AUA census data. J Urol 2016;94:195.
15. Loughlin KR. The confluence of the aging of the American population and the aging of the urological

workforce: the parmenides fallacy. Urol Pract 2019; 6:198–203.

16. Sukhu T, Pruthi NR, Deal A, et al. Workforce characteristics in urology. Urol Pract 2018;5:150–5.

17. Bhatt NR, Morris M, O'Neil A, et al. When should surgeons retire? Br J Surg 2016;103:35–42.

18. U.S. Department of Health and Human Services, Health Resources and Services Administration, National Center for Health Workforce Analysis: national and regional projections of supply and demand for surgical specialty practitioners: 2013-2025. 2016. Available at: https://bhw.hrsa.gov/sites/default/files/bureau-health-workforce/data-research/surgical-specialty-report.pdf. Accessed August 14, 2020.

19. Williams TE Jr, Satiani B, Thomas A, et al. The impending shortage and the estimated cost of training the future surgical workforce. Ann Surg 2009;250:590–7.

20. Pruthi RS, Neuwahl S, Nielsen ME, et al. Recent trends in the urology workforce in the United States. Urology 2013;82:987–93.

21. Anon: urology residency match statistics. American Urological Association 2020. Available at: https://www.auanet.org/education/auauniversity/for-residents/urology-and-specialty-matches/urology-match-results. Accessed August 6, 2020.

22. Gaither TW, Awad MA, Fang R, et al. The near-future impact of retirement on the urologic workforce: results from the American Urological Association census. Urology 2016;94:85–9.

23. Gonzalez CM, McKenna P. Challenges facing academic urology training programs: an impending crisis. Urology 2013;81:475–9.

24. Menendez R (d-N: Resident Physician Shortage Reduction Act of 2019. Available at: https://www.congress.gov/bill/116th-congress/senate-bill/348#:~:text=%202F06%202F2019)-,Resident%2020Physician%2020Shortage%2020Reduction%2020Act%2020of%20202019,fiscal%2020year%2020for%2020five%2020years. Accessed August 7, 2020.

25. Mitchell KA, Spitz A. Use of advanced practice providers as part of the urologic healthcare team. Curr Urol Rep 2015;16:62.

26. Langston JP, Duszak R Jr, Orcutt VL, et al. The expanding role of advanced practice providers in urologic procedural care. Urology 2017;106:70–5.

27. Swanton AR, Alzubaidi AN, Han Y, et al. Trends in operating room assistance for major urologic surgical procedures: an increasing role for advanced practice providers. Urology 2017;106:76–81.

28. Chen M, Kiechle J, Maher Z, et al. Use of advanced practice providers to improve patient access in urology. Urol Pract 2019;6:151–4.

29. Lajiness MJ, Quallich SA. Executive summary: standardized office cystoscopy training for advanced practice providers in urology. Urol Nurs 2020;40:31.

30. Quallich S, Lajiness S, Kovarik J, et al. Standardized office cystoscopy training for advanced practice providers in urology. Urol Pract 2020;7:228–33.

31. Langston JP, Orcutt VL, Smith AB, et al. Advanced practice providers in U.S. urology: a national survey of demographics and clinical roles. Urol Pract 2017; 4:418–24.

32. Cohen AJ, Ndoye M, Fergus KB, et al. Forecasting limited access to urology in rural communities: analysis of the American urological association census. J Rural Health 2020;36:300–6.

33. American Urological Association, Urologists in Training, Residents and Fellows in the United States 2019 Linthicum, Maryland, U.S.A., June, 2020.

34. MacQueen IT, Maggard-Gibbons M, Capra G, et al. Recruiting rural healthcare providers today: a systematic review of training program success and determinants of geographic choices. J Gen Intern Med 2018;33:191–9.

35. Helland LC, Westfall JM, Camargo CA Jr, et al. Motivations and barriers for recruitment of new emergency medicine residency graduates to rural emergency departments. Ann Emerg Med 2010;56:668–73.

36. Williams TE, Satiani B, Christopher Ellison E. A comparison of future recruitment needs in urban and rural hospitals: the rural imperative. Surgery 2011;150:617–25.

37. Shively EH, Shively SA. Threats to rural surgery. Am J Surg 2005;190:200–5.

38. Maganty A, Sabik LM, Sun Z, et al. Under treatment of prostate cancer in rural locations. J Urol 2020; 203:108–14.

39. Sadowski DJ, Geiger SW, Mueller GS, et al. Kidney cancer in rural illinois: lower incidence yet higher mortality rates. Urology 2016;94:90–5.

40. Odisho AY, Cooperberg MR, Fradet V, et al. Urologist density and county-level urologic cancer mortality. J Clin Oncol 2010;28(15):2499–504.

41. Chu S, Boxer R, Madison P, et al. Veterans Affairs telemedicine: bringing urologic care to remote clinics. Urology 2015;86:255–61.

42. Hollander JE, Carr BG. Virtually perfect? Telemedicine for Covid-19. N Engl J Med 2020;382:1679–81.

43. Gadzinski AJ, Gore JL, Ellimoottil C, et al. Implementing telemedicine in response to the COVID-19 Pandemic. J Urol 2020;204:14–6.

44. Barnes H, Richards MR, McHugh MD, et al. Rural and nonrural primary care physician practices increasingly rely on nurse practitioners. Health Aff 2018;37:908–14.

45. Hall MK, Kennedy Hall M, Burns K, et al. State of the national emergency department workforce: who provides care where? Ann Emerg Med 2018; 72:302–7.

46. American Urological Association. AUA consensus statement on advanced practice providers. Maryland: Linthicum; 2013.

47. Halpern JA, Al Hussein Al Awamlh B, Mittal S, et al. International medical graduate training in urology: are we missing an opportunity? Urology 2016;95: 39–46.

48. Opoku ST, Apenteng BA, Lin G, et al. A comparison of the J-1 visa waiver and loan repayment programs in the recruitment and retention of physicians in rural nebraska. J Rural Health 2015;31:300–9.

49. Doty B, Zuckerman R, Borgstrom D. Are general surgery residency programs likely to prepare future rural surgeons? J Surg Educ 2009;66:74–9.

50. Mercier PJ, Skube SJ, Leonard SL, et al. Creating a rural surgery track and a review of rural surgery training programs. J Surg Educ 2019;76:459–68.

51. Washington SL 3rd, Baradaran N, Gaither TW, et al. Racial distribution of urology workforce in United States in comparison to general population. Transl Androl Urol 2018;7:526–34.

52. Shantharam G, Tran TY, McGee H, et al. Examining trends in underrepresented minorities in urology residency. Urology 2019;127:36–41.

53. Vemulakonda VM, Sorensen MD, Joyner BD. The current state of diversity and multicultural training in urology residency programs. J Urol 2008;180:668–72.

54. Dai JC, Agochukwu-Mmonu N, Hittelman AB. Strategies for attracting women and underrepresented minorities in urology. Curr Urol Rep 2019;20:61.

55. Hall WJ, Chapman MV, Lee KM, et al. Implicit racial/ethnic bias among health care professionals and its influence on health care outcomes: a systematic review. Am J Public Health 2015;105(12):e60–76.

56. Orom H, Semalulu T, Underwood W 3rd. The social and learning environments experienced by underrepresented minority medical students: a narrative review. Acad Med 2013;88:1765–77.

57. Leslie Kane MA: Medscape physician compensation Report 2020. Medscape 2020. Available at: https://www.medscape.com/slideshow/2020-compensation-overview-6012684#14. Accessed August 18, 2020.

58. Nam CS, Daignault-Newton S, Herrel LA, et al. The future is female: urology workforce projections from 2020 to 2060. Sep 3;S0090-4295(20)31045-1. https://doi.org/10.1016/j.urology.2020.08.043

59. Accreditation Council for Graduate Medical Education: data resource book academic year 2018-2019.; 2019. Available at: https://www.acgme.org/About-Us/Publications-and-Resources/Graduate-Medical-Education-Data-Resource-Book. Accessed August 20, 2020.

60. Spencer ES, Deal AM, Pruthi NR, et al. Gender differences in compensation, job satisfaction and other practice patterns in urology. J Urol 2016;195:450–5.

61. Porten SP, Gaither TW, Greene KL, et al. Do women work less than men in urology: data from the American Urological Association census. Urology 2018; 118:71–5.

62. Saltzman A, Hebert K, Richman A, et al. Women urologists: changing trends in the workforce. Urology 2016;91:1–5.

63. Han J, Stillings S, Hamann H, et al. Gender and subspecialty of urology faculty in department-based leadership roles. Urology 2017;110:36–9.

64. Awad MA, Gaither TW, Osterberg EC, et al. Gender differences in promotions and scholarly productivity in academic urology. Can J Urol 2017;24:9011–6.

65. Oberlin DT, Vo AX, Bachrach L, et al. The gender divide: the impact of surgeon gender on surgical practice patterns in urology. J Urol 2016;196: 1522–6.

66. Scott VCS, Lerner LB, Eilber KS, et al. Re-evaluation of birth trends and pregnancy complications among female urologists: have we made any progress? Neurourol Urodyn 2020;39:1355–62.

67. Lerner LB, Baltrushes RJ, Stolzmann KL, et al. Satisfaction of women urologists with maternity leave and childbirth timing. J Urol 2010;183:282–6.

68. Gomez LE, Bernet P. Diversity improves performance and outcomes. J Natl Med Assoc 2019;111:383–92.

69. Marrast LM, Zallman L, Woolhandler S, et al. Minority physicians' role in the care of underserved patients: diversifying the physician workforce may be key in addressing health disparities. JAMA Intern Med 2014;174:289–91.

70. Cohen JJ, Gabriel BA, Terrell C. The case for diversity in the health care workforce. Health Aff 2002;21: 90–102.

71. Mason BS, Ross W, Ortega G, et al. Can a strategic pipeline initiative increase the number of women and underrepresented minorities in orthopaedic surgery? Clin Orthop Relat Res 2016;474: 1979–85.

72. Nellis JC, Eisele DW, Francis HW, et al. Impact of a mentored student clerkship on underrepresented minority diversity in otolaryngology-head and neck surgery. Laryngoscope 2016;126:2684–8.

73. Agawu A, Fahl C, Alexis D, et al. The influence of gender and underrepresented minority status on medical student ranking of residency programs. J Natl Med Assoc 2019;111:665–73.

74. Sharma G, Sarma AA, Walsh MN, et al. 10 recommendations to enhance recruitment, retention, and career advancement of women cardiologists. J Am Coll Cardiol 2019;74:1839–42.

75. Carnes M, Devine PG, Baier Manwell L, et al. The effect of an intervention to break the gender bias habit for faculty at one institution: a cluster randomized, controlled trial. Acad Med 2015;90:221–30.

76. North AC, McKenna PH, Fang R, et al. Burnout in urology: findings from the 2016 AUA annual census. Urol Pract 2018;5:489–94.

77. Shanafelt TD, Balch CM, Bechamps GJ, et al. Burnout and career satisfaction among American surgeons. Ann Surg 2009;250:463–71.

78. Cheng JW, Wagner H, Hernandez BC, et al. Stressors and coping mechanisms related to burnout within urology. Urology 2020;139:27–36.

79. Shanafelt TD, Balch CM, Bechamps G, et al. Burnout and medical errors among American surgeons. Ann Surg 2010;251:995–1000.

80. Dyrbye LN, Massie FS Jr, Eacker A, et al. Relationship between burnout and professional conduct and attitudes among US medical students. JAMA 2010;304:1173–80.

81. Shanafelt TD, Hasan O, Dyrbye LN, et al. Changes in burnout and satisfaction with work-life balance in physicians and the general US working population between 2011 and 2014. Mayo Clin Proc 2015;90:1600–13.

82. Kane L. Medscape national physician burnout & suicide report 2020: the generational divide. Medscape 2020. Available at: https://www.medscape.com/slideshow/2020-lifestyle-burnout-6012460#8. Accessed August 5, 2020.

83. Imran A, Calopedos R, Habashy D, et al. Acknowledging and addressing surgeon burnout. ANZ J Surg 2018;88:1100–1.

84. Pulcrano M, Evans SRT, Sosin M. Quality of life and burnout rates across surgical specialties: a systematic review. JAMA Surg 2016;151:970–8.

85. Pruthi NR, Deal A, Langston J, et al. Factors related to job satisfaction in urology. Urol Pract 2016;3:169–74.

86. Shanafelt TD, Dyrbye LN, Sinsky C, et al. Relationship between clerical burden and characteristics of the electronic environment with physician burnout and professional satisfaction. Mayo Clin Proc 2016;91:836–48.

87. Anon: World Health Organization Coronavirus Disease Dashboard. World Health Organization. Available at: https://covid19.who.int/?gclid=CjwKCAjwnK36BRBVEiwAsMT8WOAaE-vScK3BMtzuxBYLRRqXjHZanAjTTdIC5A-G-8LThBx_HYroSRoC9kAQAvD_BwE. Accessed August 30, 2020.

88. Cutler DM, Nikpay S, Huckman RS. The business of medicine in the era of COVID-19. JAMA 2020;323(20):2003–4.

89. Puliatti S, Eissa A, Eissa R, et al. COVID-19 and urology: a comprehensive review of the literature. BJU Int 2020;125:E7–14.

90. Collaborative C. Global guidance for surgical care during the COVID-19 pandemic. Br J Surg 2020;107:1097–103.

91. Katz EG, Stensland KD, Mandeville JA, et al. Triaging office based urology procedures during the COVID-19 pandemic. J Urol 2020;204:9–10.

92. Goldman HB, Haber GP. Recommendations for tiered stratification of urological surgery urgency in the COVID-19 era. J Urol 2020;204:11–3.

93. American Urological Association: COVID-19 Urology Impact Survey.; 2020. Available at: https://www.auanet.org/covid-19-info-center/covid-19-info-center. Accessed September 1, 2020.

94. Rosen GH, Murray KS, Greene KL, et al. Effect of COVID-19 on urology residency training: a nationwide survey of program directors by the Society of Academic Urologists. J Urol 2020. https://doi.org/10.1097/JU.0000000000001155.

95. Luciani LG, Mattevi D, Cai T, et al. Teleurology in the time of Covid-19 pandemic: here to stay? Urology 2020;140:4–6.

96. Ljungqvist O, Nelson G, Demartines N. The post COVID-19 surgical backlog: now is the time to implement enhanced recovery after surgery (ERAS). World J Surg 2020. https://doi.org/10.1007/s00268-020-05734-5.

97. Tachibana I, Ferguson EL, Mahenthiran A, et al. Delaying cancer cases in urology during COVID-19: review of the literature. J Urol 2020. https://doi.org/10.1097/JU.0000000000001288. 101097JU0000000000001288.

98. Khullar D, Bond AM, Schpero WL. COVID-19 and the financial health of US hospitals. JAMA 2020. https://doi.org/10.1001/jama.2020.6269.

# An Updated Review on Physician Burnout in Urology

Jennifer Nauheim, MD, Amanda C. North, MD*

## KEYWORDS

• Burnout • Professional • Health promotion • Mindfulness • Urology

## KEY POINTS

- Physician burnout is highly prevalent and starts as early as medical school.
- Burnout has an impact on the quality of life of health care workers in the United States.
- Physicians experiencing work/home conflicts are at increased risk for burnout and, although this has an impact on both male physicians and female physicians, female physicians are more affected.
- COVID-19 will very likely have an impact on physician burnout, which will reveal itself in time.
- Understanding physician burnout is important for the future of the urologist workforce, because an aging patient population already has increased the need for urologists.

## INTRODUCTION/HISTORY/DEFINITIONS/BACKGROUND

Physician burnout first was defined in 1980 by Dr Herbert J. Freudenberger as "The extinction of motivation or incentive, especially where one's devotion to a cause or relationship fails to produce the desired results."[1] Physician burnout is characterized by a triad of emotional exhaustion—a chronic state of physical and emotional depletion resulting from excessive job and/or personal demands and continuous stress; depersonalization—the development of a negative, cynical attitude toward patients; and decreased sense of personal accomplishment—a sense that work is not meaningful or important.[2] Most studies evaluating physician burnout use the Maslach Burnout Inventory (MBI), which is a 22-question validated survey using a 7-point Likert scale. Although burnout may be defined by an elevation in any of the 3 subcategories of the MBI, it usually is restricted to excessive elevations in either emotional exhaustion or depersonalization.

Urologists became more aware of the problem of physician burnout with the publication of a 2014 Mayo Clinic study[3] looking at physician burnout in the United States. Overall, physicians showed an alarming increase in the incidence of burnout compared both to the general population and to an earlier, 2011, study of physician burnout. The incidence of burnout went from 45.5% in 2011% to 54% in 2014. More worrisome for the urologic community were data showing urology as one of the worst specialties in terms of physician burnout and in term of satisfaction with work-life balance, with 63.6% of urologists in the study reporting burnout. This was a substantial increase over the 2011 study, where 41.2% of urologists reported burnout.[3] Concern over the high level of burnout in urology led to the inclusion of the MBI on the 2016 American Urological Association (AUA) Census. The overall burnout rate among urologists who participated in the Census was 38.8% but went up to 41.3% when urologists over than age 65 were excluded. There were no gender differences in burnout, perhaps due to

Department of Urology, Montefiore Medical Center, 1250 Waters Place, Bronx, NY 10461, USA
* Corresponding author.
*E-mail address:* ANorth@montefiore.org
Twitter: @JenniferNauheim (J.N.); @anorth21 (A.C.N.)

Urol Clin N Am 48 (2021) 173–178
https://doi.org/10.1016/j.ucl.2021.01.003
0094-0143/21/Published by Elsevier Inc.

the small percentage of female respondents. Working more—whether defined as more hours per week or seeing more patients per week—resulted in more burnout.[4] A follow-up study of physician burnout done by the Mayo Clinic in 2017 showed the overall rate of physician burnout had decreased to 43.9% and burnout rates in urology had decreased to 48.4%.[5]

In addition to these large, peer-reviewed studies, Medscape publishes an annual report on physician burnout. The first report to include physician burnout was released in 2013 and reported that 41% of urologists were experiencing burnout. This put urology as the eighth most burnt out specialty.[6] In 2015, burnout rates among urologists increased to 48%, which was the tenth worst specialty for burnout.[7] In 2019, the burnout rate had increased to 54%, which was well above the overall physician burnout rate of 44%, and in 2020 the burnout rate stayed at 54% whereas the overall physician burnout rate decreased to 41% (these data was published before the COVID-19 pandemic hit the United States).[8] One caution about using the Medscape data is that urologists make up a small proportion of overall respondents—with 150 of fewer urologists responding annually—which may lead to selection bias.

The 2017 AUA Census explored career regret among practicing urologists. Only 70.3% of urologists were satisfied with their career, 83.2% were satisfied with the amount of autonomy they had, and 84.5% would choose medicine as a career again. Of those who would choose medicine again, 93.4% would choose urology as their specialty.[9]

Physician burnout begins long before training is complete. Medical students start experiencing physician burnout even before graduation. A study of 4402 medical students found that 49.6% were experiencing burnout, 58% screened positive for depression, and 9.3% reported suicidal ideation in the past year. The medical students were more likely to report emotional exhaustion (41.1%) than depersonalization (27.2%). Burnout seems to increase with each subsequent year of medical school before peaking in third year and then declining slightly in fourth year.[10]

An Association of American Medical Colleges (AAMC) study showed that physician burnout worsened in residency but depression and suicidal ideation improved; 50% of residents experienced burnout, 50.7% screened positive for depression, and 8.1% reported suicidal ideation in the past year.[11] Other studies have shown high levels of burnout among residents from various specialties. One study evaluating 665 surgical residents found that 69% of them met the criteria for burnout, with

female surgical residents having a burnout rate of 73%.[12] When looking at internal medicine residents at the beginning of training compared with the end of internship, Ripp and colleagues[13] found that burnout rates increased dramatically. At the start of training, the burnout rate was 36% but had increased to 81% by the end of intern year. Among those who started internship free from burnout, 75% developed burnout by the end of the year.[13]

A 2018 *JAMA* article compared burnout rates among residents in various specialties and found that urology residents fared poorly; 63.8% of postgraduate year 2 (PGY-2) urology residents reported burnout, with 15.5% reporting career decision regret.[11] Looking only at urology residents, Machalik and colleagues[14] found that 68.2% of respondents reported burnout, with no gender differences in burnout. Burnout decreased as the residents progressed through their training.[14] The 2019 AUA Resident and Fellow Census explored burnout and career regret among urologic trainees; 82.9% of residents and 92.8% of fellows said that they would choose medicine as a career again. Male residents and male fellows were more likely to choose medicine again compared with women (84.6% of male residents vs 78.7% of female residents and 94.0% of male fellows vss. 90.0% of female fellows). Of those who would choose medicine again, 95.9% of residents and 94.4% of fellows would choose urology again. Only 48% of residents said that they never had considered another career during training. PGY-2 was the year mostly likely to report reconsidering career choice, with 28.3% of PGY-2s questioning their choice, whereas chief residents were unlikely to question their career choice with only 1% reporting rethinking their career choice. Physician burnout was reported in 47.0% of urology residents, with PGY-2s having the worst burnout at 65.2% and chief residents having the least burnout at 40.0%.[9]

It would be naïve to not consider the impact of COVID-19 on burnout among urologists. Many physicians were deployed to COVID-19 units and many practices have had to shift toward telehealth. One chief urology resident described her experiences in being deployed to the COVID-19 units in New York City at the height of the pandemic: "I would be lying if I said there was not any fear on my part as it is natural to fear the unknown. There were rumors that several residents had gotten sick with at least 1 fellow resident in another New York City program actually dying of the virus."[15] As discussed previously, rates of burnout decrease as residents progress through their surgical training; however, the impact that

COVID-19 and redeployment will have on resident burnout remains to be seen.

The pandemic also brought with it a sudden shift in the way many physicians were forced to practice medicine in a very short time. In an article by Watts and colleagues,[16] converting a practice to telemedicine in order to avoid freezing the practice was discussed. This was done by 1 of the largest hospital networks in the United States. This posed a particular challenge due to health care disparities leading to higher death rates and rates of contracting the virus. Difficulties with this transition included lack of reliable Internet access, language barriers, and reimbursements from the Centers for Medicare & Medicaid Services (CMS). CMS did pass a waiver that modified the rules surrounding telemedicine, allowing for reimbursements regardless of the location where the visit occurred and allowing for reimbursements for audio-only telemedicine.[16] Adapting to new ways of practicing medicine may have an impact on physician burnout and need to be studied further.

## DISCUSSION

Physician burnout has been shown to be related to lack of autonomy, long work hours, lack of control of work schedule, financial issues, feeling isolated, inefficient and/or hostile work environments, and setting unrealistic goals or having them imposed on oneself.[17] Like residents, attending urologists have more burnout when they work more. The AUA Census data found that working more clinical hours per week, working more overall hours per week, or seeing more patients per week all increased burnout. Midcareer urologists (those in practice 10–25 years) have more burnout than early career urologists.[9] In other fields of medicine, this increased burnout has been correlated to increased workload in midcareer physicians.[18]

Working more led to more burnout among urologic trainees also. In the Machalik and colleagues study, working more than 80 hours per week and/or having difficult to access or unavailable mental health services worsened burnout. Reading for pleasure, spending time with family/friends, and having access to mental health services all improved burnout.[14]

Satisfaction with work-life balance worsened for physicians overall between 2011 and 2014.[3] Work-life balance improved in 2017 but did not reach 2011 levels.[5] Work-life imbalance has been correlated with burnout in other specialties. In 1 study of general surgeons, those with a recent conflict between work and home were more likely to experience burnout. In this study, 47% of surgeons reported a recent work/home conflict.

Risk factors were younger age, female gender, having children, and working more hours per week.[18]

The 2017 AUA Census inquired about work-life balance for practicing urologists. Overall, 67.3% said that work left them enough time for family and personal life; however, there was a gender divide, with 68.2% of male urologists reporting that they have enough time for family and personal life and only 57.6% of female urologists reporting enough time for family and personal life. Female urologists aged 45 and under reported the worst work-life balance, with a meager 36.3% reporting enough time for family and personal life. Other major causes of workplace dissatisfaction included electronic medical records (EMRs), decreasing reimbursements, and CMS mandates.[9]

Much of the literature on burnout prevention has focused on physician self-care. Things like preventative health maintenance, exercise, proper sleep and nutrition, mindfulness meditation, and appropriate mental health care fall into this category. Many physicians are resistant to mental health services. There is a fear of licensing repercussions for seeking mental health care, which acts as a barrier.[19] Given that burnout and depression often are comorbid, counseling has been shown to decrease emotional exhaustion and sick leave at 1-year follow-up.[20] Participation in a stress management program has been shown to decrease medication errors and malpractice claims.[21]

Mindfulness teaches individuals nonreactive awareness of their affective response to external events and is important in changing the internal experience of stress. It is characterized by nonjudgmental, sustained, moment-to-moment awareness of physical sensations, perceptions, affective states, thoughts, and imagery. Health care professionals have been shown to benefit from mindfulness even more so than the general population.[22]

Several national organizations offer support to help physicians cope with burnout. The AUA was able to assess burnout among its membership by including the MBI in the 2016 AUA Census.[9] The goal was not only to better understand the impact of burnout in urology in order to offer assistance to urologists but also to present these data to organizations like the CMS to demonstrate the impact of new regulations on physicians. The AUA is using a multiprong approach to burnout: help for urologists with burnout through education, political advocacy to help politicians and government organizations understand the impact of policy on burnout, and practical solutions, such as the AUA Quality (AQUA) Registry, to give urologists a way of complying with new regulations.[23]

The American College of Graduate Medical Education (ACGME) is recognizing that burnout is a major problem during residency. At the 2016 ACGME Annual Educational Conference, burnout was included on the program and the slides made publicly available on the ACGME Web site as a webinar. Burnout and suicide prevention are important topics for the ACGME, and there are multiple webinars available on their Web site. Their goal is to include physician wellness training in residency programs nationally and increase awareness about the risks of burnout and suicide during residency.[24]

Some of the best work on burnout prevention and suicide prevention comes from the American Medical Association (AMA). The AMA has created the STEPS Forward program, which offers many helpful modules. These modules are divided by topic: patient care, workflow and process, leading change, professional well-being, and technology and finance. Workflow modules can help physicians increase efficiency in their practices whereas suicide prevention modules may help save physician lives.[25]

Over the past several years, women have entered medical school at a rate that exceeds men for the first time in history. Although urology has been slower to catch up with the gender trends in medicine, the number of women urologists has increased over time. According to the 2019 urology residency match statistics, of 389 applicants, 101 were female, with a match rate of 83%. This was an improved match rate over 2018 when 106 females applied out of 402 total applicants, with a match rate of 79%.[26] Due to the low number of female respondents, the 2016 AUA Census was unable to show increased burnout in women urologists[9]; however, most studies on physician burnout show that female physicians experience more burnout than male physician. It is likely that future studies on physician burnout in urology will show this gender difference as women make up a greater percentage of the urologic workforce.

The way medicine is practiced will forever be changed by the impact of COVID-19. This has had an impact on health care workers on every level, and the long-term effects on mental health and physician burnout will reveal themselves in time. This has affected urologists at both the attending and resident levels. Attendings in some hospitals were forced to convert all office visits to telemedicine visits to assess and triage scheduled and newly referred patients. Although there are numerous benefits to this new realm of medicine, there are strains as well, including Internet access, language barriers, and difficulties obtaining reimbursements. Some urology resident physicians were deployed to medicine COVID-19 floors. One study distributed a survey to 144 residency programs with a 45% response rate. Reserve staffing had started in 80% of programs. Redeployment was reported by 26% of programs; 60% of programs reported concern that residents will not meet case minimums due to COVID-19.[27] The fear associated with the unknown and social media postings about residents succumbing to the virus likely will cause a negative impact among resident physicians. Many residency programs have tried to adapt. The educational model for residents has evolved in the era of COVID-19 with many lectures series online, providing residents with access to education and information in ways not previously seen. The flexibility of online lectures could be beneficial to residents, allowing them to learn on their own time. With increased didactics and lectures, however, come increase stress. Residents who are off service taking care of COVID-19 patients may not have the emotional energy to dedicate to education. The challenges faced by residents fearing for their personal safety and the safety of their loved ones may foster an environment for learning. Program leaders are encouraged to hold recurring forums for residents to acknowledge and discuss their daily challenges. Health care systems should consider regular house staff screenings for psychiatric conditions, including anxiety, depression, insomnia, and distress; mental health services, including emergency hotlines, should be readily available to those in need.[28]

## SUMMARY

Physician burnout is an issue having an impact on the practice of medicine in the United States. Burnout begins in medical school and worsens during residency training. PGY-2 urology residents are at the highest risk of burnout among urology residents. Estimated rates of physician burnout among practicing urologists has ranged from approximately 38% to well above 60%. Although burnout is not synonymous with depression, the 2 can be comorbid and, therefore, physicians experiencing burnout need to have access to well-being programs and mental health care. Just knowing that mental health services were available was enough to reduce burnout in urology residents.

Work-life imbalance is a cause of practice dissatisfaction and may be a risk factor for physician burnout. Female gender and younger age both increase the risk of conflict between work and home life. As the number of women entering the field of urology increases, these young urologists will need support and mentorship to help navigate work-life balance. Changes in medical practice also may have an impact on physician burnout. The requirement to use EMRs has become a major practice dissatisfier for urologists. Increasing government regulation and decreasing reimbursements also have led to dissatisfaction with medical practice. Helping physicians improve workflow and participating in political advocacy may be 2 ways to mitigate these issues.

Although self-care is important for mental and physical well-being, it does not address many of the underlying causes of physician burnout. Urologists should be encouraged to practice self-care—regular medical visits, destigmatized mental health care, healthy diet, routine exercise, and mindfulness meditation are all important components of a healthy lifestyle. These acts of self-care alone will not prevent frustration from loss of autonomy, practice inefficiencies, and other changes in our health care system. Self-care needs to be promoted while still promoting improvements in practices.

Finally, it is hard to process the impact that COVID-19 has had on physicians' experiences. From coping with uncertainty and loss to permanent changes in health care delivery, fully understanding the long-term effects of this pandemic is awaited. COVID-19 has accelerated telemedicine practically overnight, with changes in requirements for billing and reimbursement. This may be a positive outcome of the pandemic. But many urologists and urology residents who served on the frontlines may suffer lasting negative effects from seeing loss and devastation first hand. There also have been financial hardships to both private practice urologists as well as employed urologists from decreased surgical volume and patient volume while communities were in lockdown. Whether this impact is lasting or not remains to be seen.

## DISCLOSURE

The authors have nothing to disclose.

## REFERENCES

1. Freudenberger HJ, Richelson G. Burnout: the high cost of high achievement. Garden City: Doubleday; 1980.
2. Maslach D, Jackson S, Leiter M. Maslach burnout inventory manual. 3rd edition. Palo Alto (CA): Consulting Psychologists Press; 1996.
3. Shanafelt TD, Hasan O, Drybye LN, et al. Changes in burnout and satisfaction with work-life balance in physicians and the general US working population between 2011 and 2014. Mayo Clin Proc 2015;90: 1600.
4. North AC, McKenna PH, Sener A, et al. Burnout in urology: findings from the 2016 AUA annual census. Urol Prac 2018;5(6):489.
5. Shanafelt TD, West CP, Sinsky C, et al. Changes in burnout and satisfaction with work-life balance in physicians and the general US working population between 2011 and 2017. Mayo Clin Proc 2019;94:1681.
6. Review, 2013 Lifestyle Report, et al. Medscape 2013 Physician Lifestyle Report. Available at: www.medscape.com/sites/public/lifestyle/2013. Accessed February 6, 2020.
7. Latest Medical News, Clinical Trials, Guidelines - Today on Medscape. Available at: www.medscape.com/slideshow/lifestyle-2015-overview-6006535. Accessed February 6, 2020.
8. Latest Medical News, Clinical Trials, Guidelines - Today on Medscape. Available at: www.medscape.com/slideshow/2019-lifestyle-urologist-6011153. Accessed February 6, 2020.
9. Available at: https://www.auanet.org/research/research-resources/aua-census/census-results. Accessed February 6, 2020.
10. Obregon M, Luo J, Shelton J, et al. Assessment of burnout in medical students using the maslach burnout inventory-student survey: a cross-sectional data analysis. BMC Med Educ 2020;20(1):376.
11. Drybye LN, Burke Se, Hardeman RR, et al. Association of clinical specialty with symptoms of burnout and career choice regret among US resident physicians. JAMA 2018;320:1114.
12. Hutter MM, Kellogg KC, Ferguson CM, et al. The impact of the 80-hour resident workweek on surgical residents and attending surgeons. Ann Surg 2006; 243:864.
13. Ripp JJ. The incidence and predictors of job burnout in first-year internal medicine residents: a five-institution study. Acad Med 2010;85:1304.
14. Machalik D, Brems J, Rodriguez A, et al. The impact of institutional factors on physician burnout: a national study of urology trainees. Urol 2019;131:27.
15. Davuluri M. Urology chief resident turned medicine intern: experience during the covid-19 new york city pandemic. J Urol 2020;204(4):638–9.
16. Watts KL, Abraham N. Virtually perfect for some but perhaps not for all: launching telemedicine in the bronx during the COVID-19 pandemic. J Urol 2020;204(5):903–4.
17. Balch CM, Freischlag JA, Shanafelt TD. Stress and burnout among surgeons: understanding and managing the syndrome and avoiding adverse consequences. Arch Surg 2009;144:371.
18. Dyrbye LN, Freischlag J, Kaups KI, et al. Work-home conflicts have a substantial impact on career decisions that affect the adequacy of the surgical workforce. Arch Surg 2012;147:933.

19. Rath KS, Huffman LB, Phillips GS, et al. Burnout and associated factors among members of the Society of Gynecologic Oncology. Am J Obstet Gynecol 2015;213:824.

20. Rø KE, Gude T, Tyssen R, et al. Counselling for burnout in Norwegian doctors: one year cohort study. BMJ 2008;337:a2004.

21. Jones JW, Barge BN, Steffy BD, et al. Stress and medical malpractice: organizational risk assessment and intervention. J Appl Psychol 1988;73:727.

22. Johnson JR, Emmons HC, Rivard RL, et al. Resilience training: a pilot study of a mindfulness-based program with depressed healthcare professionals. Explore (NY) 2015;11:433.

23. Available at: https://www.auanet.org/practice-resources/aua-quality-(aqua)-registry. Accessed February 6, 2020.

24. Available at: https://www.acgme.org/Portals/0/PDFs/Webinars/July_13_Powerpoint.pdf. Accessed February 6, 2020.

25. Available at: https://edhub.ama-assn.org/steps-forward. Accessed February 6, 2020.

26. Available at: https://www.auanet.org//education/auauniversity/for-residents/urology-and-specialty-matches. Accessed February 6, 2020.

27. Rosen GH, Murray KS, Greene KL, et al. Effect of COVID-19 on urology residency training: a nationwide survey of program directors by the Society of Academic Urologists. J Urol 2020;204(5):1039–45.

28. Kwon YS, Tabakin AL, Patel HV, et al. Adapting Urology Residency Training in the COVID-19 Era. Urology 2020;141:15–9.

# Development of Physician Leaders

Laura Crocitto, MD, MHA[a],*, Deepak A. Kapoor, MD[b], Kevin R. Loughlin, MD, MBA[c]

## KEYWORDS

- Physician • Leadership • Medical education • Diversity

## KEY POINTS

- Physician leadership in health care.
- Physician leadership training.
- Physician culture.
- Leadership principles.

## INTRODUCTION

Health care today is rapidly evolving and so too must health care leadership. Many external forces, including the implementation of the Affordable Care Act, have resulted in a transition of health care systems away from the traditional fee-for-service (FFS) models and toward value-based care. This has led to increasing pressures on the system to improve access, affordability, and quality.[1] These external forces are also impacting the physician workforce resulting in high physician burnout and attrition. Added to this is a rapidly changing health care environment with new technologies and treatments continuously becoming available and an aging population with increased complex care needs. Together these factors have resulted in a need for new care delivery models that emphasize team-based care. Change requires the engagement and cooperation of many different stake holders including physicians. Health care leaders must be equipped to work in this complex and rapidly evolving environment. Currently, most health systems are run by nonphysician hospital administrators. Given the significant challenges facing health care today strong and expert leadership is needed. Physicians, naturally viewed as leaders, are especially suited to this role for their expertise clinically and their credibility with other physicians. This is also true of independent medical practices. Although larger single-specialty and multispecialty groups may have the economic ability to retain business executives as managers, for many smaller groups, particularly those facing economic challenges, this burden typically falls on a practicing physician. Traditional physician leaders lack the formal training in many of the skills that are required for our current leaders, yet they have many of the necessary skills required to be successful. Growing our physician leader workforce requires formal training of existing physician leaders and a modification of the current medical school curriculum to ensure that there are qualified physician leaders in the pipeline ready and able to continue this work going forward.

## WHY PHYSICIAN LEADERS

Historically, hospitals were run primarily by physicians. This practice has decreased over the past 80 years such that now only about 5% of US hospitals are run by chief executive officers (CEOs) with a medical degree.[2] Recent evidence suggests that hospitals with strong physician leadership may perform better in terms of quality of care, physician engagement, and cost efficiency. In 2019, greater than half of the 21 US News and

a Cancer Services, UCSF Medical Center, Helen Diller Family Comprehensive Cancer Center, 1825 4th Street, L6103C, San Francisco, CA 94158, USA; b Integrated Medical Professionals, Solaris Health Holdings, LLC, The Icahn School of Medicine at Mount Sinai, 340 Broadhollow Road, Farmingdale, NY 11735, USA; c Vascular Biology Research Laboratory, Boston Children's Hospital, 300 Longwood Avenue, Boston, MA 02115, USA
* Corresponding author.
*E-mail address:* laura.crocitto@ucsf.edu

Urol Clin N Am 48 (2021) 179–186
https://doi.org/10.1016/j.ucl.2021.01.002

World Report "Best Hospitals" were managed by physician CEOs.[2,3] Further analysis demonstrated that quality scores in physician-run hospitals were 25% higher than in nonphysician-led hospitals.[2] In the United Kingdom, hospitals with more physicians in management roles scored 20% higher on financial and clinical quality scores.[2] According to the Centers for Medicare and Medicaid services, in 2018, physician-led accountable care organizations led the Medicare Shared Savings Program in net savings per capita compared with nonphysician-led accountable care organizations.[4] Although the data are suggestive only, it does provide support for the move toward increasing the presence of physician leaders in health care.

Physician leadership may be important for the quality and financial success of health systems, but it may also be critical for hospitals and independent practices struggling with physician burnout. Hospital CEOs recognize burnout as one of the most significant factors affecting health care today.[5] In 2014, 54% of physicians had one symptom of burnout, which is two times the general US population.[6] Burnout has been shown to lead to an increase in the rate of medical errors, poorer clinical outcomes, decreased productivity, and lower patient satisfaction.[6] Burnout ultimately results in physicians leaving the workforce before retirement age contributing to a national growing physician shortage. In urology, burnout is especially high with 54% of urologists reporting burnout compared with 42% of physicians overall.[7] Many of the factors that give rise to physician burnout including increased administrative burdens and the use of an electronic health record are out of the control of administrators and leaders. Engagement, however, which is viewed as the opposite of burnout, is one factor that leaders may have some influence over.[8] In 2016, according to Gallop, 33% of employees on average were engaged at work.[9] Engaged employees are less likely to suffer burnout and less likely to leave the job.[10]

Research has shown that supervisors who have expertise in the field are linked to increased company performance and employee satisfaction across industries including sports, education, and medicine.[11] Increasing the presence of physician leaders can improve physician engagement. In medicine, physicians respect the voice of other physicians as someone who has "walked the walk" and has knowledge of what occurs on the front lines. Thus, physician leaders, with their deep understanding of the core business, have the advantage of having greater credibility with other physicians and ultimately improving engagement.[12,13] Physician leadership is important for

addressing burnout and critical to the future of health care.

## LEADERSHIP AND DIVERSITY

Promotion and growth of a physician leader workforce must include promotion and growth of diversity within this workforce. Diverse leadership teams are associated with improved medical quality, reduced health care disparities, and improved financial outcomes.[14,15] It is estimated that by 2043, most of the population will be comprised of racial and ethnic minorities. This is currently reflected in the increasing diversity of the patient population. As these demographics change, it will be important to ensure diversity at all levels of the workforce including in leadership and board composition.[16] Today, minorities make up 32% of the patient population while holding only 11% of executive leadership roles.[2,17] In fact, more than 90% of all hospital CEOs are White (non-Hispanic, or Latino).[18] Additionally, women who make up slightly more than 50% of the population, half of the workforce, and hold 50% of the doctoral degrees are also scarce in leadership roles. In fact, only 18% of health care CEOs are women and only 3% of the C-suite roles are held by minority women.[18,19] Even with evidence to suggest the benefits of women leaders on financial performance, risk, social responsiveness, and firm value, women still advance to leadership roles at a much lower rate than men.[19] Today roughly 50% of medical students are women yet only 38% of full-time medical school faculty are women, 21% full professors, 15% department chairs, and 16% deans.[20,21] In urology 30% of incoming residents are women, yet only 3.3% of department chairs are women verses 14% of department chairs across all specialties.[21] A focused effort to address diversity and equity in the workplace is important if we want to decrease the disparities seen in minority patient care, improve the quality of life of the workforce, and increase profitability.[22,23]

## CHANGING HEALTH CARE ENVIRONMENT

Since the enactment of the Affordable Care Act in March 2010, health care organizations have found themselves in the midst of significant external pressures. Hospital systems are now being rewarded for delivering high-quality, patient-centered, coordinated care at reduced costs. There is a shift from FFS to value-based care. There is an increased emphasis on public health and the wellness of populations. This is being driven through shared risk arrangements, capitation, and bundled payment strategies requiring significant redesign of clinical care models.[24,25] Hospitals and health systems have had to build the information technology infrastructure to comply with meaningful use, which promotes the electronic exchange of health information. Quality public reporting brings transparency to hospital outcomes but requires a significant investment in data infrastructure and quality-improvement efforts. Patients are increasingly more informed and empowered as consumers of health care driving changes in practices around access, cost, and choice of care. Reimbursements continue to decrease and there is increasing competition for these limited dollars in the market.[25] The population is aging and requires more complex health care in the face of a projected shortfall of up to 139,000 physicians by 2033.[26] Currently, a large proportion of the physician workforce is reaching retirement age, and this may be accelerated because of effects of burnout and the COVID-19 pandemic. All of these changes in the health care industry require fundamental changes in the way health systems interact with physicians.[27] Strong leaders are needed to drive these changes in health care delivery and to lead the physicians through this change.

Physicians are facing similar challenges and external pressures as health care systems including the need to adapt to new payment models, decreasing reimbursements, the costs of implementing an electronic health record, and building the infrastructure to meet the quality reporting requirements. These external forces are driving physicians to join larger groups or become employed by hospital systems. In 2018, 47% of practicing physicians in the United States were employed, whereas 45.9% owned their practices. This was the first time that the number of employed physicians exceeded the number who owned their practices. The number of physicians who worked directly for a hospital or work in hospital-owned practices was 34.7%, up from 29% in 2012.[28] As physicians transition from self-employment to employed status they struggle with a loss of autonomy, which is a fundamental aspect of the physician culture. Physicians also face increasing administrative burdens. This includes the growing need for prior authorizations by insurance companies, increasing documentation requirements, increased burden of pay for performance initiatives, increasing maintenance of certification requirements, and increased consumerism of medicine with no obvious connection to improved patient outcomes. This along with the recent COVID-19 pandemic is resulting in increased physician burnout and may ultimately drive many physicians to an early retirement at a time when there is an increasing demand for providers to care for an aging and complex population.[29]

The cumulative results of these external pressures on the health care system is meant to drive change from the traditional FFS system to a value-based system. Significant change must occur over the next decade to fully implement value-based care. This current environment presents an important opportunity for physician leaders to combine their clinical background with leadership skills. In this way, physician leaders can help other practitioners understand novel payment models in a distinct and different way at a time when strong "expert" leadership is needed.[30] The American College of Physician Executives includes physician leadership as one of its nine essential elements required to provide optimal patient-centered care. The organization believes that, to succeed, health care must be quality-centered, safe, streamlined, measured, evidence-based, value-driven, innovative, fair and equitable, and physician-led.[31]

## PHYSICIAN LEADERS

Traditional physician leaders were chosen based on their credentials, seniority, clinical competency, and political standing.[1] One's individual legacy as a clinician, educator, and researcher was valued above all else when selecting a physician leader. This practice begins with the intense socialization process of physician training. The health profession is founded on a rigorous scientific discipline that values autonomous decision making, personal achievement, and the importance of improving one's own performance rather than that of an institution.[1,27] Medical schools value and encourage individuals who look to self, not others, for answers. Consequently, physicians are often put into leadership roles based on their standing as a respected physician in their field. This model was successful when physician leaders were expected to be advocates for resources and liaisons between administrators and other physicians.[27] As we continue to evolve, the skills required to be a successful physician leader are changing and may not now be the same skills required to be an effective physician. To address the gap in skills between traditional physician leaders and more formally trained physician leaders, health systems often pair physicians with an administrator. The dyad leadership model has been important for the growth of traditional physician leaders but can also hinder physician leaders when administrators step in to fill the skill gaps verses mentoring and ultimately empowering the physicians to acquire these skills themselves. Furthermore, although institutional and larger independent providers may have the resources to support this model, this is much more complicated for smaller groups. The current climate calls for strong physician leaders with high emotional intelligence, knowledge of the business of health care, formal leadership training, and team building skills in addition to their clinical acumen and professional standing.[17]

This transformation may be particularly challenging for independent groups. In urology, as increasing numbers of physicians are institutionally employed, a simultaneous trend is the formation of large urology-centric groups; by 2016, such groups provided more than a third of the nation's urologic care.[32] These groups typically coalesce around individual physicians who use a charismatic model of leadership; this model relies on "their ability to communicate in a moving, emotionally charged way. By expressing their visions with power and inspiring trust, they influence those they lead and persuade them into action."[33] Once formed, effecting change may require completely different skills than that required to actuate formation of the group[34]; engagement of different stakeholders and delegating authority may be a challenge for physicians accustomed to a more top-down leadership structure. The anthropologic concept of liminality, which describes an intermediate state in a rite of passage, appropriately describes the transition between clinician and administrator.[35] Physicians in this liminal state face challenges in which their leadership roles and needs of the institution may not be completely consistent with their historical personal goals; understanding how to modify their historical individual use of power to a more distributed model is key to this transition.[36]

Transitioning from a physician to a physician leader is challenging in other ways. As physicians move into administrative positions they work more closely with administrative leaders. Historically, there has been a large cultural divide between physicians and administrators resulting in distrust between the two.[37] Physicians come from an expert culture in which its members are cohesive and have a highly developed personal identity. The culture is based on biomedical sciences and the scientific method. Physicians rely on hard facts and are suspect of soft data. They typically have minimal exposure to the business side of health care. Their focus is on the individual patient with physicians viewing themselves as the champions of patient care. They assume that resources are unlimited and should be available to all to maximize quality. They work autonomously and are experts at problem solving, working under pressure, and rapid decision making.[38]

The administrative culture, however, is one built on social and management sciences. It has a collective focus with the group valued over the individual. Administrators use soft qualitative data and have a loose professional identity. They embrace organizational values, missions, and visions. Decision making is usually team based. Most have minimal exposure to health care professionals or front-line clinical care. They focus on populations verses the individual patients. They view themselves as the protector of the hospital where resources are limited and so allocated appropriately.[38]

As physicians move into leadership roles, it is important to understand the cultural differences along with the new skill requirements that one needs, which is a source of frustration in the new role. The transition from physician to physician leader requires a shift from technical competence and clinical expertise to more soft skills, such as team building and relationship building. Physician leaders must leave the command and control methods behind in favor of a more collaborative style.[30] They must move from acting to visioning and strategizing. The pace of change at the system level is often much slower than with clinical care. Challenges are often not clearly defined, and without an obvious solution. There is a need to approach problems in a team-based manner, which can lead to anxiety around the dependance on others. There may be a loss or changes in old relationships with colleagues and peers and challenges in forming new ones. As the physician transitions into the administrative role they can often be viewed by their colleagues as "going to the dark side" or becoming a suit. Administrators are also often weary of physicians, viewing them as the reason for the high costs of care. This can lead to a questioning of one's professional identity. There may be a lack of self-confidence in the new role as they begin the transition.[37] It is important for health systems to be aware of these challenges and provide continued support for these physicians as they move into their leadership roles.

Physicians inherently have many of the qualities needed in leaders. They are fast learners, outcome driven, comfortable with responsibility and decision making, have high expectations, and an unparalleled work ethic.[30] That being said, they often need to modify the way they approach things and at the same time acquire new skills. Professional organizations, including the American Association for Physician Leadership, formerly the American College of Physician Executives, have created a list of some 300 competencies needed in a physician leader. They grouped them into five primary areas: (1) knowledge of the health care environment, (2) professionalism, (3) communication and relationship management, (4) business skills and management, and (5) leadership.[2,30]

## TRAINING PHYSICIAN LEADERS

Urologic leaders, like urologic surgeons, are not born. They are made by years of training. However, traditionally there has been little leadership training in medical school, residency, or throughout most urologic careers. In addition, there are physicians in practice who are moving into leadership roles and thus, we must be able to provide education at all points in one's career. Current medical school curricula are beginning to incorporate basic leadership training, but it is not universal, and the methodology varies from institution to institution. There is no consensus or data to determine the best method for teaching leadership, the areas to be taught, or the timing of the coursework. Most of the courses are taught by clinical faculty, and most are taught in an isolated fashion, not longitudinal over time.[39] Medical school curricula are often already impacted and some programs are even shortening the training to 3 years making it even more difficult to incorporate a formal leadership program. It is recognized, however, that even early in one's training there is a need for trainees to work collaboratively across disciplines, lead teams, and train and mentor those in junior positions.[39] Medical schools should consider selecting medical students with the desired leadership qualities by putting more emphasis on the human and interpersonal skills on the Medical College Admission Tests and entrance criteria. They need to be encouraged to offer leadership modules, at least as electives, in the last year of medical school, which can then be continued throughout training and beyond. During residency, there should be lectures on the elements of leadership and required reading assignments. Three skills that all physician leaders require are (1) to speak well, (2) to write well, and (3) basic business acumen. Residency program directors need to provide opportunities throughout training for residents to acquire these skills. In the same manner that residents receive feedback on their surgical and clinical skills, there should be formal feedback on their leadership development.

Leadership training should not cease at the time of residency graduation. The American Urological Association offers a well-structured and valuable leadership program that is available to American Urological Association members; Large Urology Group Practice Association and the American Association of Colleges & Universities offer topic-specific programs to enhance physician management skills knowledge base. Many universities offer truncated executive business training programs and some individuals may opt to enroll in formal master's in business administration or master's in public health programs.

Currently, there are some programs that offer an MD and a formal master's in business administration degree together.[12,37] Some professional organizations offer postgraduate opportunities, such as the American Association for Physician Leadership and American College of Healthcare Executives, and many institutions, such as Mayo Clinic and the Cleveland Clinic, offer their own in-house programs.[2,39] The most successful programs incorporate a formal curriculum on the business of health care and leadership skill with mentorship and coaching by role models in addition to experiential learning in progressive leadership roles.

## LEADERSHIP ROLES FOR UROLOGISTS

Urologic leadership takes on many roles. It is not limited to roles within the medical profession. Although within academic urology obvious leadership positions include chairpersons and program directorships, in private practice urology leaders are needed as managing directors. Other urologists will serve as chief medical officers, CEOs, or, in some cases, deans. Other leadership opportunities include editorial positions and serving on hospital and medical school committees.

In addition to the formal positions outlined previously, urologists use leadership training every day in practice. When a urologist is in the operating room or in clinic, he or she is leading a team where leadership training has tangible applications.

Finally, physicians are respected leaders in their community and their fellow citizens often look to them for guidance on a variety of topics. It is not unusual to observe urologists on school boards and town councils or as authors on op-ed and other newspaper articles. Urologists should be aware that leadership has many faces. Nowhere has the opportunity for civic leadership been more apparent than in the recent COVID-19 crisis.

## WHAT MAKES A GOOD LEADER?

Although leadership styles differ, there are seven traits that are common to leaders.[40]

1. *Integrity*. Integrity is the most important leadership quality. Former Wyoming senator, Alan K. Simpson summed it up best, "If you have

integrity, nothing else matters. If you don't have integrity, nothing else matters."

2. *Vision*. In the rapidly changing field of urology, vision is a quality that is essential for a leader. Vision facilitates the establishment of priorities, allocation of resources, and strategic planning.

3. *Be a Good Listener*. Beware of those who interrupt. Not only do good listeners show respect for their colleagues, they learn by listening. Good listeners are good students. The corollary to being a good listener is being a good observer. Tom Peters, the Stanford management guru said, "You can learn a lot by just walking around."[41]

4. *Humility*. Many surgeons do not like to use the words, "I don't know." Not only are these important words for a surgeon, they are particularly important for a surgical leader. Humility, rather than a weakness, actually empowers the leader. Hubris is not a leadership quality. Those who consider themselves the smartest person in the room are invariably not.

5. *Persuasion Not Power*. The surgical world engenders ad hoc pronouncements. Although, at times, the leader must mandate a policy, often arbitrary, the effective leader looks at the long game. If policies and decisions are arrived at by persuasion, by consensus, that leader banks future credibility and trust, which is invaluable.

6. *Avoid Isolation*. Many leaders, either by position or temperament, become isolated. This is a dangerous circumstance for a leader. A good leader should encourage a coterie of close advisors who he or she can trust. A leader needs to have someone who will say directly, "I think you are wrong." In her book, *Team of Rivals*,[42] the presidential historian Doris Kearns Goodwin emphasized that one of the qualities that made Abraham Lincoln such a great leader was his ability to value the opinions of those who disagreed with him.

7. *Arrogate Not, Be Unselfish*. It is easy for those in power to unfairly take credit for accomplishments that were not their own. Most academic urologists have observed senior faculty arrogating the accomplishments of junior faculty or residents. When this occurs, it severely undermines morale and any spirit of teamwork and unselfishness, which are critical components of good leadership.

## HOW ARE UROLOGIC LEADERS SELECTED?

The short answer to this question is in too many cases, the selection is arbitrary and not thoughtful. An individual with a lengthy curriculum vitae or a robust grant history may be given a leadership position without either the temperament or experience to function as an effective leader. The same traits that contributed to the publication and research accomplishments do not necessarily translate into leadership skills. The chairperson or professor who continues to be primarily focused on their own ongoing achievements, often neglects the time and energy required to lead and mentor others. Mature leaders realize before accepting a leadership position that it is necessary to put many of their own goals on hold. A hallmark of a good leader is one who is amplified by the accomplishments of their colleagues, rather than be threatened by them. Too often that is not the case.

One of the strengths of our profession has been the emerging role of women and minorities. This presents our specialty with a challenge and an opportunity. Leadership training needs to be modified to train a more diverse constituency. Women, in particular, have already made enormous contributions to the world outside of medicine. Of 195 countries, 70 have had women leaders and females occupy almost 20% of Congressional seats.[43] Medical schools and health systems must invest in flexibility policies (job sharing, part-time work) and faculty development and mentoring.[20] Organizations must make a concerted effort to hire women and minorities.

To continue to be leaders in health care delivery and advance urology, the talent pool needs to be expanded beyond White men. Diversity has the potential to be urology's greatest strength. The increasing influence of female urologists and the greater representation of diverse ethnicities and cultures serve to better populate leadership resources and to better serve the multicultural population of the United States.

## EMOTIONAL INTELLIGENCE, THE UNDERPINNING OF LEADERSHIP

In 1995, Goleman[44] published his landmark book, *Emotional Intelligence*, which has been part of most business school curricula ever since. In it, he argues that emotional intelligence is as important as IQ for success. He identifies the elements of emotional intelligence as self-awareness, self-regulation, motivation, empathy, and social skills.[44] These characteristics are the underpinning of leadership. As urologists, it should be our goal to develop these qualities in ourselves and in those who we identify as our future leaders. The mantra for urologic leaders was captured by Bill Gates when he said, "As we look ahead into the next century, leaders will be those who empower others."

## CLINICS CARE POINTS

- The rapidly evolving health care environment is resulting in an increased need for leaders with clinical expertise and strong business acumen. This is driving many health care systems to hire and develop physician leaders with formal business training.

- Increasing diversity at all levels of the health care workforce is needed to decrease health care disparities. Additionally, increased diversity within leadership has been shown to improve medical quality and financial outcomes.

- The transition from a physician to a physician leader often requires that the physician acquire a strong business knowledge of health care, and develop their leadership skills with an emphasis on emotional intelligence and team building.

- Physician leadership training should begin in medical school and continue throughout their training and into their careers.

- Physicians are often viewed as natural leaders. Building on this with formal training in the business aspects of health care, urologists can and should take on leadership roles within their practice or health system and within their community.

## DISCLOSURE

The authors have nothing to disclose.

## REFERENCES

1. Stoller JK. Developing physician-leaders: a call to action. J Gen Intern Med 2009;24(7):876–8.
2. Gupta A. Physician versus non-physician CEOs: the effect of a leader's professional background on the quality of hospital management and health care. J Hosp Adm 2019;8(47). https://doi.org/10.5430/jha.v8n5p47.
3. Goodall AH. Physician-leaders and hospital performance: is there an association? *Soc Sci Med* 2011;73(4):535–9.
4. Gonzalez-Smith J, Bleser WK, Muhlestein D, et al. Medicare ACO results for 2018: more downside risk adoption, more savings, and all ACO types now averaging savings. Health Aff Blog 2019. https://doi.org/10.1377/hblog20191024.65681.
5. Physician burnout is a public health crisis: a message to our fellow health care CEOs. Health Aff Blog 2017;28. https://doi.org/10.1377/hblog20170328.059397.
6. Han S, Shanafelt TD, Sinsky CA, et al. Estimating the attributable cost of physician burnout in the United States. Ann Intern Med 2019;170(11):784–90.
7. Kane L. Medscape national physician burnout & suicide report 2020: the generational divide. Medscape 2020.
8. Henson JW. FACHE reducing physician burnout through engagement. J Healthc Manag 2016;61(2):86–9.
9. Gallup. State of the American Workplace. 2017. Available at: https://www.gallup.com/workplace/238085/state-american-workplace-report-2017.aspx.
10. Rao S, Ferris TG, Hidrue MK, et al. Physician burnout, engagement and career satisfaction in a large academic medical practice. Clin Med Res 2020;18(1):3–10.
11. Goodall AH. Should doctors run hospitals? In: Dice Report. 2013. Available at: http://ifo.de/docdl/dicereport113-forum7.pdf. Accessed October 25, 2020.
12. Turner J. Why healthcare C-suites should include physicians. In: Managed Healthcare Executive. 2019. Available at: http://managedhealthcareexecutive.com/view/why-healthcare-c-suites-should-include-physicians. Accessed September 17, 2020.
13. Stoller JK, Goodall A, Baker A. Why the best hospitals are managed by doctors. In: Harvard Business Review. 2016. Available at: http://hbr.org/2016/12/why-the-best.hospitals-are-managed-by-doctors. Accessed September 30, 2020.
14. Dotson E, Nuru-Jeter A. Setting the stage for a business case for leadership diversity in healthcare: history, research, and leverage. J Healthc Manag 2012;57(1):35–46.
15. Feyes E. Leadership and the promotion of diversity in the work force and beyond. In: PressBooks. Available at: http://ohiostate.pressbooks.pub/pubhhmp6615/chapter/leadership-and-the-promotion-of-diversity-in-the-work-force-and-beyond/. Accessed September 18, 2020.
16. Henkel G. Does U.S. healthcare need more diverse leadership? 2016. In: The Hospitalist. Available at: https://www.the-hospitalist.org/hospitalist/article/121639/does-us-healthcare-need-more-diverse-leadership. Accessed September 18, 2020.
17. Athey LA. Why healthcare leaders need to take a new look at diversity in their organizations. Chicago: ACHE; 2015.
18. Diversity and disparities: a benchmarking study of U.S. hospitals in 2015. American Hospital Association; 2015. Available at: https://www.aha.org/system/files/hpoe/Reports-HPOE/diversity_disparities_chartbook.pdf.
19. Chisholm-Burns MA, Spivey CA, Hagemann T, et al. Women in leadership and the bewildering glass ceiling. Am J Health-System Pharm 2017;5(74):312–24.

20. Winkel AF. Every doctor needs a wife: an old adage worth reexamining. Perspect Med Educ 2019;8(2): 101–6.

21. Han J, Stillings S, Hamann H, et al. Gender and subspecialty of urology faculty in department-based leadership roles. Urology 2017;110:36–9.

22. Hunt V, Layton D, Prince S. Diversity matters. McKinsey & Company; 2015. Available at: https://www.mckinsey.com/business-functions/organization/our-insights/~/media/2497d4ae4b534ee89d929cc6e3aea485.ashx.

23. Gomez LE, Bernet P. Diversity improves performance and outcomes. J Natl Med Assoc 2019; 111(4):383–92.

24. Antos JR, Capretta JC. The future of delivery system reform. Health Aff Blog 2017. https://doi.org/10.1377/hblog20170420.059715.

25. Young GJ. Hospitals in the post-ACA era: impacts and responses. In: The Milbank Quarterly. 2017. Available at: https://www.milbank.org/publications/hospitals-post-aca-era-impacts-responses/. Accessed October 20, 2020.

26. AAMC. (2020). New AAMC report confirms growing physician shortage. Available at: https://www.aamc.org/news-insights/press-releases/new-aamc-report-confirms-growing-physician-shortage.

27. Atchison TA, Bujak JS. Leading transformational change: the physician-executive Partnership. 1st edition. Chicago: Health Administration Press; 2001.

28. Kane CK. American Medical Association. Policy research perspectives: updated data on physician practice arrangements: for the first time, fewer physicians are owners than employees. 2018. Available at: https://www.ama-assn.org/system/files/2019-07/prp-fewer-owners-benchmark-survey-2018.pdf.

29. Kane L. "US and international physicians' COVID-19 Experience Report". Medscape 2020.

30. Angood P, Birk S. The value of physician leadership. Physician Exec 2014;40(3):6–20.

31. Angood PB. Changing demographics, competencies and physician leadership. Chicago, IL: AHA Physician Alliance; 2013.

32. Shore ND, Kapoor DA, Goldfischer ER, et al. Preserving independent urology: LUGPA's first decade. Rev Urol 2019;21(2–3):102–8.

33. 5 types of leadership styles in healthcare. Advent Health University Healthcare Blog. 2020. Available at: https://online.ahu.edu/blog/leadership-styles-in-healthcare/. Accessed October 16, 2020.

34. Garfield J. Leading change: what is being asked of physician leaders? American Association for Physician Leadership. 2018. Available at: https://www.physicianleaders.org/news/leading-change-what-being-asked-physician-leaders. Accessed October 16, 2020.

35. Hazelton L. Crossing the threshold: physician leadership and liminality. Can J Phys Leader 2017;4: 47–9.

36. Saxena A, Meschino D, Hazelton L, et al. Power and physician leadership. BMJ Leader 2019;3:92–8.

37. Bhardwaj A. Alignment between physicians and hospital administrators: historical perspective and future directions. Hosp Pract (1995) 2017;45(3): 81–7.

38. Fiol CM, O'Connor EJ. Separately together: a new path to healthy hospital-physician relations. 1st Edition. Chicago: Health Administration Press; 2009.

39. Sultan N, Torti J, Haddara W, et al. Leadership development in postgraduate medical education: a systematic review of the literature. Acad Med 2019;94(3):440–9.

40. Loughlin KR. Surgical leadership. In: Mansfield C, editor. Leadership in thought, word and deed. Morrisville, NC: Lulu Publications; 2019. p. 42–50.

41. Peters T, Watermen PH. In search of excellence; lessons from America's best run companies,1982, Harper Business Essentials

42. Kearns Goodwin D. Team of rivals. the political genius of Abraham Lincoln. New York: Simon and Schuster; 2006.

43. People facts. Available at: https://facts.net/history/people/women-leaders-facts. Accessed October 1, 2020.

44. Goleman D. Emotional intelligence: why it can matter more than IQ. New York: Bantam Books; 1995.

# Women in Urology

Mara R. Holton, MD*, Kari Bailey, MD[1]

## KEYWORDS

- Female urologist • Woman urologist • Pay discrepancies • Gender disparities • Breastfeeding
- Maternity leave

## KEY POINTS

- The demographic trend of GU training presages a significant increase in the slope of the shift toward female representation in GU clinical practice in the next decade.
- There are significant differentials within clinical practice between men and women, including selection of subspecialization, practice milieu, and practice geography.
- Women in GU continue to experience discrimination and harassment and also have unique challenges, including assumptions about gender roles, accommodations for pregnancy and breastfeeding, along with pay disparities.
- GU has extant provider workforce shortages, which will likely worsen, particularly in rural areas, based on current patterns of female postgraduate training and selection of clinical practice environment.
- In order for the field of GU to evolve and adapt to the demographic trends, the differences in training and practice experiences between men and women should continue to be identified and addressed.

## HISTORY

The role of certain women as caretakers for the sick and injured has assuredly existed since the beginning of cooperative human society. There is abundant historical evidence that women have participated in maternal and neonatal care, particularly to facilitate labor and provide assistance immediately after parturition. Peseshet (c. 2500 BCE), "lady overseer of the female physicians," may have been responsible for training midwives at an ancient school in Egypt.[1] Medical texts from the library at Ashurbanipal in the ancient Assyrian empire demonstrate that midwives, *sabsutu*, were routinely in attendance at births, and the records from the Greeks have several references to women practicing both Obstetrics and Gynecology as well as more general medical care.[2] Nonetheless, although notable exceptions exist beyond reproductive care, as specialization within society evolved to create formal roles for those who treated ailments of all types, the historical record suggests that most of these earliest dedicated providers of health care were men.

Certainly, the pathologic condition of the genitourinary (GU) tract has contributed to human misery since antiquity. Evidence of detailed anatomic study of the GU tract and uroscopy as a diagnostic tool is replete in the historical record. Furthermore, the existence of early urologic subspecialization is exemplified by Hippocrates' familiar admonition from the fifth century BCE, "...to leave such [urologic] procedures to the practitioners of that craft."[3] As medical and surgical training became more formalized throughout the middle ages, women were systematically and specifically excluded from participation outside of a very limited purview. In fact, beginning in the Middle Ages, the characterization of women with any medical knowledge as witches,[4] combined with the rigorous exclusion of women from increasingly structured medical education, consigned those few remaining to practice only in limited capacities and in total obscurity.

AAUrology, PA, Annapolis, MD, USA
[1] Present address: 600 Ridgely Avenue, Suite 213, Annapolis, MD 21401.
* Corresponding author. 600 Ridgely Avenue, Suite 213, Annapolis, MD 21401.
*E-mail address:* mholton@aaurology.com

Urol Clin N Am 48 (2021) 187–194
https://doi.org/10.1016/j.ucl.2020.12.003

## EVOLUTION

These entrenched attitudes and assumptions regarding the female role in the provision of health care finally began to reverse, only haltingly, close to a millennium later. It was ultimately through tremendous resourcefulness, perseverance, and even the sheer serendipity of mistake that, despite Osler's assessment that admitting women to medical school had been a "failure," he was forced to concede that the "die was cast" in the late nineteenth century.[5] However, notwithstanding this tentative and partial step of women in the United States into the field of medicine during the industrial revolution in the late 1800s, it was believed that women did not need and were not capable of receiving the same scientific education as their male counterparts. There was fear that the study of certain aspects of medicine, including anatomy, would damage a woman's character or lead them astray sexually. For that reason, women were not permitted to dissect male genitalia and were given castrated papier-mâché models.[6] Upon examining this early modern history of women in medicine, it is apparent why women's clinical representation in GU lagged well into modern days and is particularly notable for its languorous pace compared with that of many other medical fields. Although unable to receive equivalent education and training to participate in the field of urology, some women were nonetheless able to innovate technology and theory to advance the field. In 1878, Anna Broomall, a surgeon at the Women's Hospital of Philadelphia, created a lithotrite that was attached to a dental drill to break large bladder calculi.[6] In addition, in the late 1800s, Mary Putnam Jacobi, a physician, scientist, and advocate for women's rights, published in The Lancet on the theory of urethral syndrome.[6]

By the 1920s and 1930s in the United States, several determined women were entering into formal urologic training. Dr Mary Child MacGregor trained in urology at the New York Infirmary in 1928 and went on to become the Chief of Urology at that institution. She was a mother of 2 and fostered babies who were put up for adoption. Unfortunately, in other cases, limitations imposed by conventions regarding pregnancy and motherhood precluded a full practice.[6] Dr Rosemary Shoemaker completed a 4-year fellowship in urology at the Mayo Clinic in 1938 and had 2 daughters during her training. She was not permitted on the urologic surgery staff while pregnant and thus was relegated to spending a significant amount of her residency time studying pathologic condition. After her training was complete, she opened a clinic dedicated to the care of women and children but was unable to sustain this limited practice and eventually worked as a pathologist. Other women were similarly unable to maintain a surgical urologic practice and elected to leave the field and practice other medical specialties.[6] In other cases, discouraged from surgical urology in the mid-twentieth century, several female urologists were nevertheless able to sustain successful and durable medical urology practices.

In 1962, Elizabeth Pickett became the first female board-certified urologist. By the mid-1970s, female urologists had grown to a notable handful, gaining enough national attention that an article in Parade magazine was published highlighting women in the field.[6] By 1985, there were 22 women practicing urology in the United States, representing almost half of the only 50 female urologists practicing worldwide at that time. In a survey from that era, these women reported choosing the field for, among other things: diagnostic techniques; the combination of medicine and surgery; and favorable hours.[6] Interestingly, in surveys regarding the choices of modern trainees, these features continue to be frequently cited reasons by both men and women who choose to train in this field.[7]

## TRENDS IN MEDICAL AND UROLOGY TRAINING

The slow-moving pace of these nascent years contrasts with the exponential advancement and penetration of women into the field of urology over the last 3 decades, paralleling the overall trends of women in medical training. The last 40 years have seen staggering demographic shifts in female medical school enrollment and participation in residency spots. Although women made up less than one-quarter of medical school matriculants in 1975, in 2017, for the first time, the majority (50.9%) of US first year medical students were women. Over approximately the same period, the proportion of overall female residents increased from 15.4% to 46.1%.[8]

These trends are not, however, symmetric across all medical and surgical specialties, and women are still proportionally underrepresented in many surgical fields. According to 2017 data from the Association of American Medical Colleges (AAMC), women make up less than one-quarter of 10 surgical specialties, including urology, orthopedic surgery, thoracic surgery, and neurosurgery.[9] In the case of GU, the gender disparity has, nonetheless, narrowed over the past 15 years. American Urological Association (AUA) data from 1996 to 2015 demonstrate that the number of female applicants to urology residency programs increased from 13.6% to 25.9% over that decade and that there was a similar match rate between male and female candidates.[8] This finding translated to a 429% increase in female urology trainees over the study period, with women accounting for 22.7% of the residency trainees in 2015.[8]

## TRENDS IN CLINICAL PRACTICE

Despite these prominent shifts in female students and trainees overall, the percentage of female urologists in the United States has increased only a modicum over the last few years. In 2014, of almost 12,000 practicing urologists, only 7.7% were women; by 2019, female representation, although it had increased slightly, still represented just less than 10% of practicing urologists[10] (**Fig. 1**).

The more recent increase in female GU trainees corresponds to a predominance of comparatively younger women in clinical practice. In 2019, the AUA census demonstrated that 22% of practicing female urologists were less than 45 s old, whereas only 6% were greater than 55 years old (**Fig. 2**). This finding contrasts with their male colleagues who are, on average, 56 years old.[10] Another notable distinction between male and female urologists is the increased likelihood that female residents will pursue fellowship training and, of those, 35% will have pursued postgraduate work in pediatrics or female pelvic and reconstructive medicine.[10] This tendency toward additional postresidency training may partially contribute to the fact that women are 20% more likely than their male colleagues to choose to practice in an academic or hospital setting.

## GEOGRAPHIC OBSERVATIONS

A geographic preference for dense urban centers also distinguishes female urologists from their male colleagues in the United States. Although only 2.1% of the total urologists in the United States characterize themselves as practicing in a small town or rural setting, most practicing female urologists live and work in urban areas with a population of greater than 1 million.[11] This finding is likely related, in some degree, to the higher incidence of fellowship training by female residents and consequently greater tendency toward practice within or associated with an academic practice, as academic centers are generally located in more population-dense areas. In other cases, this may simply be related to a preference for academic centers, but it may also reflect a tendency of women trainees to select more urban locations

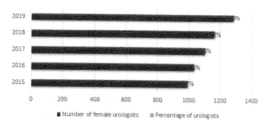

**Fig. 1.** Number and percentage of female practicing urologists, 2015 to 2019. (*Data from* American Urology Association (2019). The State of the Urology Workforce and Practice in the United States.)

for a variety of other reasons, including job opportunities for a partner.

Although it is difficult to discern which factors are causative and to what degree, the prevalence of fellowship training in tandem with predilection for urban practice location is correlated with the disproportionate representation of female providers in academic settings. There are, of course, other reasons an academic position may be compelling to women, and some reasonable suppositions include the following: (1) generally more robust benefits packages, particularly paid maternity leave benefits, which are still extraordinarily rare in the private practice setting; (2) more flexible schedules; (3) less Relative value units focus, potentially allowing for longer patient visits; (4) part-time or flexible work opportunities in academia; (5) support on-call by residents/Advanced practice providers; and (6) more collegial atmospheres in academia. Further elucidation of the relative contribution of any of these variables, along with the identification of others, is contingent on continued investigation and research.

## CLINICAL PRACTICE PATTERNS

As more women enter the GU workforce, studies have been conducted to examine practice patterns between sexes and have demonstrated a tendency toward same-sex patient care by women providers. In a study comparing surgical

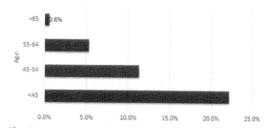

**Fig. 2.** Percentage of female practicing urologists by age. (*Data from* American Urology Association (2019). The State of the Urology Workforce and Practice in the United States.)

volume, women were more likely to perform gender-neutral procedures (ESWL, TURBT, ureteroscopy) on female patients and more likely to perform female-specific surgery. Men performed more than 3 times as many vasectomies and twice as many prostatectomies as their female colleagues. In addition, female GU patients were 1.65 times more likely to be seen by a female provider than by a male provider.[12]

The presumption, commonly asserted anecdotally, that women in urology practice elect disproportionately for part-time work are not borne out by the statistics. In fact, analysis of the AUA census data in 2014 demonstrated that men and women work essentially the same number of hours on average. This finding is in contrast to the statistics for medicine as a whole, which show women work less hours than their male counterparts.[13] Distinctions between gender practice pattern do exist however, and the AUA census data demonstrated that women providers tend to have longer office visits and see fewer patients on average.[14] The relative predominance of women in practice working in academic settings may partially account for this time differential, as visits in these locations are often associated with more complex or specialized problems and average visits pers provider are typically less than in a private practice setting.

## CHALLENGES AND DISPARITIES

As the number of female medical students has increased, the male-to-female representation of trainees and clinicians within many fields has achieved equity and, in some cases, such as Obstetrics and Gynecology, female predominance. However, surgery and many surgical subspecialties continue to be dominated by male attendings and trainees. Although the most flagrant examples of discrimination are far less common than they were decades ago, it is still not unheard of for female surgical staff to find an absence of dedicated female changing facilities proximate to operating rooms or to meet bemusement when trying to obtain scrubs or gloves of the appropriate size. It is at the peril of the field of urology that it is assumed these are anachronisms, and one may fail to recognize both the cost and the frailty of the gains within surgery as a whole and GU in particular. Each advance represents the manifestation of the work of countless diligent and enlightened men and women who recognize the manifold benefits of diversity, both to patients and to their provider colleagues. It is thus critical that those factors are identified that impede progress and create barriers.

### Professional Advancement/Mentorship

As previously discussed, female urologists are more likely to practice in an academic setting and have fellowship training. However, this does not translate to similar levels of achievement in academic centers or in career advancement within academia. Breyer and colleagues analyzed the 2017 urology census to find that among academic urologists, men authored more publications and were more commonly principal investigators. It took women, on average, 1.2 years longer to advance from assistant professor to associate professor, and male colleagues had a 3 times higher rate of rapid advancement.[14] It is hypothesized that these disparities may result from underrepresentation of women in senior leadership or from women spending more time in administrative and/or teaching roles rather than research or may be associated with the disproportionate time women spend on daily family responsibilities when compared with male peers with families. In order to foster a more diverse academic environment in the future and provide meaningful opportunities for professional growth, it is critical to highlight these differences and identify and mitigate causes. As in other fields, this will require adaptation, creativity, and flexibility, and a willingness to relinquish potentially long-established customs and assumptions.

### Pregnancy, Maternity Leave, and Breastfeeding Issues

The combined features of younger age and gender will inevitably mean that pregnancies during training and practice, maternity leave, breastfeeding policies, and childcare issues will become ever more significant. Although these issues are present for both male and female providers, the biologic facts of gestation and neonate nutrition create an irrefutable disproportionate "burden" on female providers who choose to carry a pregnancy and parent young children. Furthermore, although the primary obligations of child-rearing in dual sex couples have been shifted from the exclusive domain of the female partner, there is still wide recognition that women bear most of the responsibilities related to the child or children. These issues, increasingly extant within many fields of medicine over many decades, will escalate in immediacy and relevance in GU, especially as women of childbearing and child rearing age are increasingly represented in clinical practice.

Maternity leave, or its absence, is another deterrent for women entering a surgical, maledominated field. The American Board of Urology (ABU) formally determined in 1980 that residents would *not be penalized* for taking maternity leave. However, the current leave policy states that a resident must complete at least 46 weeks per residency year to graduate, which correlates to a maximum of 6 weeks of maternity leave if no other time whatsoever is taken off. Thirty years after the first explicit pronouncement about maternity leave for GU residents, there is still no specific mention of maternity leave in the current ABU resident leave guidelines.[15] Recently, however, the American Board of Medical Specialties, which includes the ABU among its member boards, promulgated recommendations effective July 2021. These guidelines specifically reference "reasonable leaves of absence" for several reasons, including the care of a newborn, and suggest accommodations during pregnancy and lactation.[16] Although these are only recommendations, this represents a meaningful step in the ad hoc, and often punitive, nature of maternity leave.

In 2009, female urologists were surveyed to determine satisfaction with maternity leave both in and after residency. Only 42% of women reported a formal maternity leave policy during residency. Just less than one-half of the surveyed respondents had a child before completing residency (10% before residency and 38% during residency); slightly more than half (52%) of respondents did not have a child until the completion of her training. However, the timing of birth, while in or out of residency, was not a factor in dissatisfaction, rather this assessment correlated with length of leave. In both residency and in practice, most women took maternity leave for 8 weeks or less; those women who took 9 weeks or longer were *three* times as likely to report being satisfied with their duration of leave.[17]

Accompanying the challenge of absence from residency training or clinical practice during maternity leave is the continued difficulty of breastfeeding upon return to work. Barriers to establishing a breast pumping routine for physician mothers include inadequate time, schedule inflexibility, and inadequate space. A survey study of physician mothers reported longer maternity leave, dedicated space to pump, and accommodating schedules as factors contributing positively to lactation to 12 months' postpartum or to their personal goal. More than 30% of respondents reported pumping in their car, empty patient rooms, bathrooms, locker rooms, and/or closets.[18] Women in nonsurgical specialties were able to maintain lactation for a longer duration postpartum than women in surgical specialties, likely because of more inflexibility in schedule and fewer pumping accommodations for those in surgical practices.[18]

## Discrimination and Harassment

Although women continue to increase in prevalence in medical schools and in the medical profession, gender-specific challenges remain. There is implicit bias toward women in surgical specialties, as most are historically predominantly male. Women are met with concerns about the adequacy of their motivation to join the field and of their ability to succeed predicated purely on their gender. Female medical students have been dissuaded from entering into surgical fields based on the perception of obstacles to starting a family and emphasis on concern of a work-life balance, which will not be acceptable or achievable for women who desire to have a family. In addition, as highlighted in a 2006 survey of trainees, women are deterred from entering a surgical career based on the perception that "masculine" personality traits characterize those suited to be surgeons and of surgery being an "old boys' club."[19]

After overcoming the initial gender barrier to entry into the field, women may continually meet with discrimination and sexual harassment through training and practice. In a 2019 study of surgeons, 58% of female surgeons reported being harassed compared with only 25% of male surgeons. These incidences are more common in female trainees, who were more than twice as likely to experience harassment than attending physicians. Unfortunately, most incidents were not reported for fear of negative career impact or retribution.[20] In another survey of physician mothers, 78% of respondents reported that they had experienced discrimination in practice. In the same survey, 68% of respondents reported gender discrimination and 35% reported maternal discrimination. Maternal discrimination was defined as discrimination based on pregnancy, maternity leave, or breastfeeding. Maternal discrimination, in particular, correlated with a higher level of job dissatisfaction and burnout.[17]

Urology is not exempt and, in fact, may be more susceptible to experiences of sexual harassment and discrimination of women in the workplace. Because urology practice often deals with diseases of an intimate nature and involves routine examination of genitals, female physicians can find themselves in a vulnerable position for harassment by both colleagues and patients. In a separate survey of women specifically in urology, similar gender-specific challenges existed, including refusal to be seen by male patients and harassment by both male patients and male colleagues. More than two-thirds of female urologists report patient-perpetrated sexual harassment, with the most at-risk population being residents/fellows and physicians younger than 40 years old.[21]

## Pay Gap

The national pay gap between genders extends to medical professions. Adjusting for age, position, and specialty, women make, on average, $20K less than their male counterparts.[22] That number may well be a gross underestimation, as AAMC reports demonstrate that women are far more commonly represented in lower-paying specialties overall. Interestingly, declining trends in reimbursement in many specialties, such as Obstetrics and Gynecology and Pediatrics, directly mirror the increasing preponderance of female providers over the same interval. Although not conclusive, this is consistent with observations of the devaluation of equivalent work when performed by women rather than men. Further amplifying these disparities, a recent article found that pay gaps are even more prominent in surgical subspecialty practices where the physicians are predominantly men, as is likely to be the case in almost every existing GU practice. This study analyzed income data from more than 18,000 physicians in the United States over a 4-year period. In practices with equal male and female physicians, men earned 10% to 12% more than their female counterparts. However, when adjusting for practices with male dominance, the pay gap increased to 20% to 27%, depending on practice type. In private surgical practice, this translates to a staggering $150,000 pay differential for women in male-dominated practices.[23]

## HORIZON

Urology has seen tremendous innovation within clinical care for any number of conditions, spearheaded, at least partially, by the epic advancements in the treatment of benign, as well as malignant, prostate disease. Concomitantly, but perhaps not to the same degree, there has certainly been advancement in recognition of the morbidity of certain conditions uniquely related to the female population, such as classic female Stress urinary incontinence, overactive bladder, and pelvic prolapse. A large survey of greater than 1 million cases over several years demonstrated that female surgeons operated on women more frequently and did more female-specific procedures (index urologic procedures).[12] Furthermore, as previously discussed, female providers are more likely to have done a fellowship in female pelvic and reconstructive medicine. The further specialization could absolutely herald a positive trend, as increased attention is paid toward female-specific conditions affecting GU patients, translating into recognition, teaching, and innovative treatments. What factors are related to the selection of these fellowships however, and thus whether the trend will continue, is unclear. Whether this demonstrated preference reflects subtle discrimination, interest in a specialty whereby a mentor or practitioners are more likely to be women, identification or empathy with the patient population among other contributing factors is not yet well elucidated. As more women complete urology residency and consider fellowships, these trends may well shift.

There is also a perception that millennials, of either gender, seek a more equitable work-life balance than their predecessors within medicine. The total dereliction of personal or familial obligations is no longer uniformly openly demanded or lauded as evidence of commitment to a surgical pursuit. These changing trends, coupled with the prevalence of women in academic practices, and thereby typically seeing fewer patients, may exacerbate the already impending anticipated GU provider shortages. In addition, although this "modern" attitude is perhaps typical of junior staff of either gender, it can certainly be a source of disagreement and conflict with more senior partners, who are almost universally men.

In addition to the gender differential, practicing female urologists are, on the whole, almost a decade younger on average than their male colleagues, adding a further generational component to the disparities with more senior staff. Age disparity may well present practice issues beyond more customary gender distinctions pertaining to maternity leave, breastfeeding policies, and child-rearing obligations, as differences are further amplified and magnified by decades of social distraction. Areas of discordance or conflict may extend to social conventions regarding language or dress, work expectations, attitudes toward sexuality, marriage, and cohabitation, and a whole host of other concerns. Practices, although clearly not predicated on universally shared values and beliefs, may nonetheless struggle when confronted with stark differences of values and opinion in certain areas.

A well-documented demographic trend of continued concern has been the "graying" of the GU provider population and concomitant concerns about access and provider shortages as providers retire. In a urology workforce manpower study from 2013, note was made of declining supply of urologists per capita from 1981 along with the distribution of remaining providers into group practices and more urban areas.[24] Although the average age of the practicing male urologist in 2015 was 53, by 2018, the average age had increased to 56. Women in GU practice are, as noted previously, more than a decade younger, on average. Interestingly, however, women endorse an intent to retire younger than their male counterparts (65 vs 69).[10] Although this is only a prediction, it suggests that the workforce shortfall could become more pronounced over the next few decades if average overall career length is comparatively curtailed.

A chronic issue within medicine, and particularly within specialty care, is rural access. The AUA workforce report from 2019 demonstrates that almost 90% of all urologists practice in a metropolitan setting. The remaining minority, who practice in a micropolitan, small town, or rural area, is twice as likely to be older than 65 than younger than 45.[10] As discussed earlier, women GU providers are even less likely currently to practice in a "rural area." In light of overall GU provider shortages, this could exacerbate critical workforce resource shortages. Therefore, it is important to spend additional efforts to discern what has correlated with this trend and what factors impact female urologists' practice location choices.

## SUMMARY

We have been privileged to participate in GU at a time of extraordinary demographic and societal change. It is important to recall that, as urologists, we as specialists share far more in common than any divisions based on gender alone. We are each indebted to those many individuals, both men and women, who have dedicated their careers to our training and mentorship. We chose this specialty because of our common interest in and fascination with urologic pathologic condition, our dedication to the patients we treat, and our thrill at our ability to diagnose, and often, to surgically cure disease. Gender diversity creates challenges to established customs and paradigms and mandates dispassionate and rigorous analysis. We will address these challenges best with the creative thinking and innovation that characterize our specialty and that have advanced urologic care from early history to the modern surgical era.

## DISCLOSURE

No disclosure.

## REFERENCES

1. Harer WB Jr, el-Dawakhly Z. Peseshet–the first female physician? Obstet Gynecol 1989;74(6):960–1.
2. Mark JJ. Health care in ancient mesopotamia. Ancient history encyclopedia. 2014. Available at: https://www.ancient.eu/article/687/. Accessed July 12, 2020.
3. Hippocrates. Translation of Hippocrates by Loeb classical library. I-VIII. Cambridge (MA): Harvard University Press; 1923. p. 1995.
4. Minkowski WL. Women healers of the middle ages: selected aspects of their history. Am J Public Health 1992;82(2):288–95.
5. Palepu A, Herbert CP. Medical women in academia: the silences we keep. CMAJ 2002;167(8):877–9.
6. Gillespie L, Cosgrove M, Fourcroy J, et al. Women in urology: a splash in the pan. Urology 1985;25(1):93–7.
7. Jackson I, Bobbin M, Jordan M, et al. A survey of women urology residents regarding career choice and practice challenges. J Womens Health (Larchmt) 2009;18(11):1867–72.
8. Halpern JA, Lee UJ, Wolff EM, et al. Women in urology residency, 1978-2013: a critical look at gender representation in our specialty. Urology 2016;92: 20–5.
9. Haskins J. Where are all the women in surgery. 2019. Available at: https://www.aamc.org/news-insights/where-are-all-women-surgery. Accessed July 12, 2020.
10. American Urological Association. The State of the Urology Workforce and Practice in the United States 2019. Linthicum, MD: American Urological Association; 2020.
11. Saltzman A, Hebert K, Richman A, et al. Women urologists: changing trends in the workforce. Urology 2016;91:1–5.
12. Oberlin DT, Vo AX, Bachrach L, et al. The gender divide: the impact of surgeon gender on surgical practice patterns in urology. J Urol 2016;196(5): 1522–6.
13. Leigh JP, Tancredi D, Jerant A, et al. Annual work hours across physician specialties. Arch Intern Med 2011;171(13):1211–3.
14. Porten SP, Gaither TW, Greene KL, et al. Do women work less than men in urology: data from the American Urological Association Census. Urology 2018; 118:71–5.
15. American Board of Urology. Residency requirements. Available at: https://www.abu.org/residency-requirements/. Accessed July 14, 2020.
16. American Board of Medical Specialties. American Board of Medical Specialties policy on parental, caregiver and medical leave during training. 2020. Available at: https://www.abms.org/media/258004/parental-caregiver-and-medical-leave-during-training-policy.pdf. Accessed July 30, 2020.
17. Lerner LB, Baltrushes RJ, Stolzmann KL, et al. Satisfaction of women urologists with maternity leave and childbirth timing. J Urol 2010;183(1):282–6.
18. Melnitchouk N, Scully RE, Davids JS. Barriers to breastfeeding for US physicians who are mothers. JAMA Intern Med 2018;178(8):1130–2.
19. Gargiulo DA, Hyman NH, Hebert JC. Women in surgery: do we really understand the deterrents? Arch Surg 2006;141(4):405–8.

20. Nayyar A, Scarlet S, Strassle PD, et al. A national survey of sexual harassment among surgeons. Academic Surgical Congress (ASC) 2019 Abstract 85.06. Available at: https://www.asc-abstracts.org/abs2019/85-06-a-national-survey-of-sexual-harassment-among-surgeons/. Accessed July 20, 2019.

21. Uberoi P, Mwamukonda KB, Novak TE, et al. Patient perpetrated sexual harassment of urologists: a survey-based study. Urology Practice. 2020. 8(1). 155-159.

22. Spencer ES, Deal AM, Pruthi NR, et al. Gender differences in compensation, job satisfaction and other practice patterns in urology. J Urol 2016;195(2):450–5.

23. Whaley CM, Arnold DR, Gross N, et al. Practice composition and sex differences in physician income: observational study. BMJ 2020;370:m2588.

24. Pruthi RS, Neuwahl S, Nielsen ME, et al. Recent trends in the urology workforce in the United States. Urology 2013;82(5):987–93.

# Understanding the Millennial Physician

Jake Quarles[a], Jason Hafron, MD[b],*

## KEYWORDS

- Millennial • Millennial training • Millennial urologist • Millennial surgeon • Millennial residents
- Urology residents • Medical training • Medical education

## KEY POINTS

- Unique aspects of the millennial urologist require an understanding of their generation for successful training.
- The special characteristics of the millennial urologist will make their contributions to the medical field important for the progress of urology.
- Understanding what a millennial physician desires in their life and career is essential in being able to recruit and maintain competent millennial urologists.

## INTRODUCTION

Training and adapting to a person's unique characteristics are imperative for them to reach their full potential. Whether it be a single new hire or an entire generation, understanding is the first step to achieving this success. A prime example of this idea is represented by the millennial generation. Often misunderstood without others taking the time to understand, the millennial generation holds some of the most potential in the current day workforce. Breakdown based on American Urologic Association numbers identifies more than 25% of today's urology workforce being composed of individuals younger than 45 years.[1] A large portion of this is composed of millennials who currently make up the largest generation in the United States with more than 72 million individuals.[2] As the millennial population continues to age, the millennial American will often seek out care from those that represent themselves such that more people will begin searching for a millennial physician. By understanding the ideals, skills, and traits of the millennial generation, urology practices can attract these physicians and use all that they have to offer.

Attraction of offers is a key step in hiring the millennial physician. Realizing what they desire and what they require will help keep their interest. As mentioned, millennials are often misunderstood; however, this is not the case. Those same traits that many believe to be destructive are in actuality, the strongest traits that millennials have to offer. Unlocking this potential will help the millennial urologist bud into a strong, successful physician. Using this potential and applying it in their training will help them hone the skills to make change in the field of urology.

Generational identity represents both a person's place in life as well as a community of individuals born at a similar time. These groups typically share characteristics and can define their role of what it means to be American.[3] Commonly spanning 15 to 20 years, generations are surrounded by important cultural events. Millennials are commonly noted to have been born between 1981, when Generation X birth rates began to increase, and 1996, when cultural events shifted for a new generation to take place. The Millennial generation has been continuously shaped by key political, social, and economic events in their lifetime.

There are no relevant financial or commercial conflicts of interest to disclose.

[a] Michigan Institute of Urology, 130 Town Center Drive, Suite 101, Troy, MI 48084, USA; [b] William Beaumont School of Medicine, Beaumont Health, Michigan Institute of Urology, 130 Town Center Drive, Suite 101, Troy, MI 48084, USA
* Corresponding author.
*E-mail address:* hafronj@michiganurology.com

Urol Clin N Am 48 (2021) 195–202
https://doi.org/10.1016/j.ucl.2020.12.001

### Millennial Childhood

Millennials were raised during many tense world conditions (**Fig. 1**). Millennials graduated and entered the workforce while unemployment rates were at an all-time high.[4] They faced economic hardship from a young age growing up through the Great Recession of 2007.[5] Through these hardships though, millennials persevered. College costs were exponentially high yet they continue to be the most educated generation yet.[6] Many millennials enter urologic practice with significant student debt. More than half of residents have a debt of greater than $150,000. Surveys found that 24% of graduates enter residency with a debt of $300,000.[7]

Parents of millennials brought a new definition of family. Typically, with parents born from Generation X, the millennial generation experienced a focus on family. Families took trips together, spent time going out to eat, and more fathers attended births than ever before. Their parents, seen as the "latchkey" and "divorce" generation, brought new maturity to their roles, often with multiple hats serving as caregivers, coaches, and mentors.[8] Comparatively, many parents of millennials also took on the role of helicopter parenting. Although kids of previous generations had freedom to roam and experience life, parents of millennials kept a stricter watch on their kids. This eventually shaped the values and ideas that millennials hold toward authority and family structure.[6] Raised by these involved helicopter parents, millennials have been the busiest generation. Involved in activities such as sports, camps, and scouts, a millennial schedule has been micromanaged and occupied at an early age. Pressured with the stresses of a highly structured environment, millennials had little free time, another experience that makes them the way they are today.[8] Born post-computer revolution, millennials consistently had technology available to them. As digital natives, they appreciate the impact that technology has on their lives.[9]

### DISCUSSION
### Misunderstandings of the Millennial Perspective

Faced with different outlooks on life, millennials commonly see conflict with older generations. Millennials are perceived as entitled, lazy, need to be hand-held, and disloyal with authority issues.[6] The older generations who understand the millennial generations often have personal experience, as family or community members, with them.[6] Crystal Kadakia offers the expression of a 2-sided coin method to better understand and train millennials[6] (**Fig. 2**).

Lazy millennials classically are redefining productivity. Millennials see work as an equation. Even though you are putting in time, you may be less productive than those who focus what is required to achieve the goal. Working less hours does not mean work is not done well. It simply shows whether someone is willing to put in the energy for high-quality work. Having seen the classic 9 to 5 work life and the distractions that past generations have faced, millennials have redefined it. Millennials tend to work more efficiently and do not focus on hours at work but more the quality of their work product. Working undistracted for shorter time periods means higher efficiency than a full day's worth of distracted work.[6]

Seen as an entitled generation, millennials express themselves as entrepreneurial spirits. Classically observed as acting with an "I deserve this" mindset, millennials are driven by their desire to make the most of their potential. When asking for promotion or challenging work, it does not stem from a place of entitlement. It is a statement of wanting contributions professionally that millennials are already familiar with making in their personal lives. A freelance mentality allows for the application of talent and skills that they have honed and perfected their whole lives.[6]

Past generations criticize millennials as needing hand-holding. In actuality millennials desire agility.

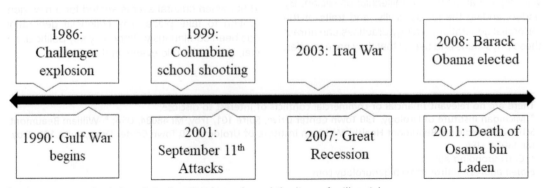

**Fig. 1.** Key events in their upbringing that have shaped the lives of millennials.

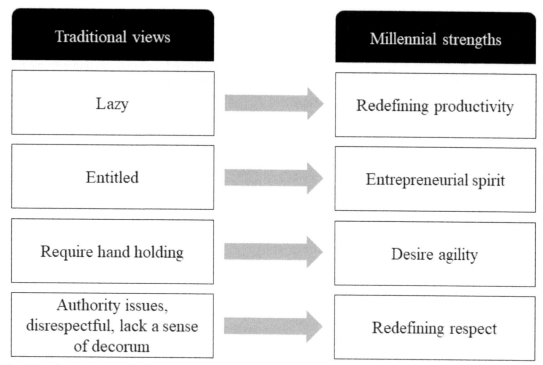

**Fig. 2.** Traditional views of millennials over camouflage millennial strengths that can serve as assets to any working team. These hidden gems in a 2-sided coin model represent all that a millennial has to offer. (*Data from* Kadakia C. The Millennial Myth: Transforming Misunderstanding into Workplace Breakthroughs. Oakland, CA: Berrett-Koehler Publishers; 2017.)

Work challenges have expanded faster than the workforce has been able to adapt to, and this creates unique and challenging scenarios placing millennials in difficult situations. Yet, gaining this information quicker and more frequently enforces agility in the working millennial. Millennials expect positive feedback from their contributions. Often seen in a negative light, this request is a way to course-correct, become agile, and succeed with limited resources.[6]

Regarded as a generation of disrespect, authority issues, and a lack of decorum, millennials serve to redefine respect.[6] From early on, millennials have had close relationships with authority figures in their life in the form of their involved and active parents. This creates relationships without the hierarchy of authority commonly seen in previous generations. Millennials may see their professors as equals and expect them to be approachable and supportive, caring for their growth similar to their parents.[10]

### The Millennial Medical Student

The training of a millennial physician begins with their medical education. Medical school applications now match the lifestyles that millennials grew up with: strong extracurricular involvement, high achievement in academics, and a major driving purpose in life. Because parents have typically been involved in their lives and the decisions they make since early on, the millennial generation has become the most accomplished generation to date with more accomplishments on their resumes in high school than previous generations have had in college.[11] With almost 80 million millennials competing in America today, numbers alone have encouraged these habits and lifestyles.[11]

### Technology

In medical school, a millennial student expects to continue learning with the technology that they have grown up on. They expect expertise and availability of this technology to enhance their learning and further prepare them for a technologically driven world. With further development of technology and its use in delivery of quality patient care, medical education can use technology to achieve its educational goals. Various simulation technologies can help accomplish these specific goals in areas of team training, critical care or trauma learning, psychomotor skill development, and enhanced decision making. Structured simulation brings together all of these skills in a safe environment and helps team building and team management for the success of both patient and practitioner.[12]

### Team-based learning

The increases seen in team-based learning (TBL) environments in medical schools is partially a response to the needs for greater social belonging in the millennial generation. These groups expect to share events, develop team instincts, and form tighter bonds that can improve the delivery of quality care.[13] Because millennials prefer an effective flexible structure and teamwork, it should not come as a surprise that students prefer a team-based learning strategy for their education.[6,14] The application and education of this sort of setup, TBL, matches the current practice of medicine as well, with teams of practitioners involved in the care of patients. The early exposure and opportunity of this sort of education provides a unique experience that millennial students may enjoy more than traditional learning. Learning this skill early on, the millennial physician will be able to improve outcomes and help their peers feel invested in their work. Studies have seen that poor teamwork has the potential and ability to not only reduce productivity, but actually damage or harm those involved in the form of burnout or depression.[15]

### Formative feedback

Formative feedback in medical education will not only encourage but will also help growth and learning. Quick immediate feedback will allow a student to course correct and will help them successfully reach their goal. Contrary to evaluation, feedback comes before this goal is reached and does not represent judgment. Feedback serves its purpose by correcting mistakes before it is too late, reinforcing good performance, and configures clinical competence.[16]

The ultimate goal is to improve the student's clinical skills. If feedback is given incorrectly it has the potential to tarnish the relationship between the mentor and student. Feedback should be given from an ally of the trainee such as a mentor or a respected superior. This feedback should be given in an appropriate setting when feedback is expected such as after a procedure or patient encounter. It should be based on experiential data and limited to behaviors that can actually be adapted or improved on. There should be minimal evaluative language, and generalization should be avoided. Subjective data can be appropriate but should be identified upfront. Feedback should focus on concrete decisions and actions rather than interpretations made by one's assessor. Finally, be wary of positive feedback and its relationship with personal praise. Putting these guidelines into practice may take time, but feedback has an important role in clinical education.[16]

### The Millennial Urology Resident

As generations change, their training and education changes as well. As changes are made to a millennial physician's education beginning with medical school, it continues with their residency and fellowship. Eventually, the attending population will be most of the millennial physicians. With this in mind, one must start the acceptance of their ideas, lifestyles, and characteristics as they begin their residency training. Although it may be difficult, it is important to allow them to share their perspective. Roles may need to be reversed. Typical attending seniority will be enhanced as they take mentorship roles with millennial residents. Allowing these millennials who were trained in medical school with new ideas, technology, and paradigms to share their perspective and guide senior physicians will be important to push forward the future of medicine.[17] Because millennials have grown up with this technology, it is important to encourage senior physicians to be accepting of their ideas and suggestions. Similarly, as attendings teach their residents, they must keep in mind the characteristics of millennials. Millennials may be accustomed to being proficient in this technology. The struggle to adapt plus their natural impatience needs to be matched by attending patience and the opportunity for prolonged training. These ingredients will allow for millennials to become adept in their training.[11]

### The importance of mentorship of the millennial urology resident

Millennials expect mirrored conduct in their attending mentors as they are mastering their skill. This means that the communication and availability should match their own. Being constantly connected through technology and messaging systems their whole lives, millennials expect to be connected this same way with their mentors. They expect fast responses, frequent availability, and short meetings to course correct and remain on task; contrary to traditional mentorship models that involve fewer but longer meetings. These millennials hope to create a team of mentors with this same mentality that are all in their corner. Believing in the power of teams and groupthink, a multidisciplinary team of mentors with different ideals and backgrounds offers the most to a rising millennial physician. As opposed to the traditionally thought of mentorship, millennials are not often bound by hierarchical boundaries. The millennial physician will seek out the most appropriate and beneficial advice, which may mean that they go over one's head or a specific mentor is not used.[17] These relationships should not discourage or upset mentors of other generations; remember that millennials are not entitled, they are entrepreneurs. They actively seek benefit and are driven by their own potential. As mentors teach and educate millennial physicians, they must keep in mind these driving factors.

### Distinctive goals of the millennial urology resident

Millennials do not derive satisfaction from traditional academic success and praise as often as their predecessors did. They often have goals and would get this satisfaction from things such as results of studies or training, implementation of their hardwork, or device and procedure development.[17] In a rapidly advancing field such as urology, millennial residents want implementation and success instead of research and trials. If they feel they have the ability to help right now, they want to put that forth and make the difference. Similar to the way that they were raised, they want to make this difference in the world. This desire can be implemented through multiple interests and avenues. They may have multiple careers and hobbies, one of which happens to be medicine. Some millennials are just now entering residency. Others may be just now beginning to consider medicine as a possible career. These nontraditional students will soon begin their path to becoming a millennial urologist.[11] The mentors and program directors of millennial residents need to be open to feedback from their residents. Similarly, to how residents expect respectful, honest, and supportive feedback, it is very much reasonable for programs and attendings to expect the same from their residents. Because of the way they were raised, millennials often have a comfortability with the authority figures in their life. This will benefit open and honest communication in both parties of their training.[10]

### Education strategies for the millennial urology resident

As the mentorship and relationships develop, millennial education will come to fruition. However, adaptations to traditional educational styles are important for millennial success. Millennials often prefer active learning in forms of interaction, workshops, simulation, and game style presentations. Traditional slide-show presentations without interaction as questions, video, or discussion are easily forgotten or ignored. The addition of slide-show presentations to flipped-classrooms or peer-to-peer teaching can reinforce ideas. Simulation, teamwork, and discussion resemble real-life scenarios and can provide a comfortability in the training of the millennial physician. The presentation of this educational material can vary as mentioned. However, millennials also expect availability of this material for their own use through accessibility to shared resources for students to learn from and use in their unique ways. Availability through senior residents and attendings is just as important in teaching as text resources are. Intergenerational styles of teaching show value in educating millennials. Senior residents are required to know the material in order to present and answer questions for their junior residents. This team-based system is accurate of a traditional residency hierarchy and ensures that people are competent in their field. This type of presentation can be improved with preassigned learning material in forms of readings, video, or podcasts and then reinforce the information with discussion during allotted time.[18]

### Millennial urology resident perception of work hours

As residency regulations change, the practicing millennial urologist may adjust their ideal working situation postresidency. When asked how many hours they felt reasonable as an attending physician, most current residents stated between 51 and 60 hours per week. This is in contrast to the new maximum requirements of 80 hours per week residents currently work. Working 51 to 60 hours per week, millennials hope to achieve the work-life balance they so much desire. This work-life desire is also reflected in the amount of call that current residents find reasonable. Most of the residents have stated that a reasonable call schedule would be 2 to 3 nights per month. However, older-generation urologists currently average 5 to 8 nights of call per month.[19] These expectations or desires by millennials are topics of discussion that need to be covered when recruiting new physicians.[19] Professional schedule and decisions need to be discussed but so do personal and livelihood discussions. Benefits will become increasingly important for millennials, especially because they focus on their families and starting their lives. College costs have gone up year after year. With loan payback often needing to be done from undergrad and medical school loans, this needs to be considered for offerings and paybacks when recruiting the millennial.[6] Family focus needs to be heavily considered as well with items such as vacation, insurance benefits, and both maternity or paternity leave. Recruiters need to have a family mindset to appeal to the millennial urologist.

## Millennial Burnout

Even with all the benefits and covered assets, urology burnout is inevitable. Urology has been noted as one of the top 5 specialties facing the highest burnout. More than half of urologists reported that they have experienced it. Currently, the generation with the greatest levels is Generation X. These doctors are trying to balance their established family lives, figure out their career trajectory, and continue planning and staying on track for retirement. This needs to be addressed, however, because these are the same problems that millennials will face in a few years' time. These millennials said that bureaucratic tasks such as charting or paperwork have contributed the most to their current and future burnout. Up to 77% of millennials have stated that this burnout has had an impact on their relationships. Coming out of an already stressful time for relationships in residency, the newly practicing millennial physician will be hit again with these threats as a practicing physician. Millennials have stated that this culmination of burnout has affected their spouses, partners, and families—all things that are very important to the millennial. More women have reported this burnout than men: up to 48% of women compared with 37% of men. Because more and more women are entering urology, this needs to be focused on to limit the detrimental effects. To cope with these feelings, 45% of physicians said they isolate themselves from others. This type of approach has a negative impact on a team-focused residency program as well as the team aspects of medicine, potentially placing patients at risk.[20]

In order to combat this burnout, committees have made efforts to promote wellness. The ACGME Council of Review Committee Residents has identified necessary tactics to combat physician burnout. Firstly, one must promote faculty and peer mentorship to enhance relationship and communication. Secondly, a supportive culture must be established, allowing for comfortability in a safe space. Thirdly, efforts must be made to destigmatize depression and recognize that burnout is occurring. Finally, programs need to create avenues to identify these depressive thoughts and allow physicians to get access to confidential resources that they need. Individual wellness committees in practices can assist in the development of physician wellness and elimination of burnout.[21]

## How to Best Incorporate the Millennial Urologist into Practice

Utilization of a millennial urologist involves providing them the tools to unlock their full potential. As digital natives, millennials expect the newest technology and the ability to apply and use these tools in their day-to-day work. Technology plays such a large part in the perception that a millennial may have about a job that 42% of millennials have said they would quit their position if they were required to work with substandard technology.[22] The application and opportunity of technology in urology is ripe for growth and exploration. New technology, in the form of imaging, diagnosis, and surgery or treatment, serves as challenges that millennials are keen on taking on. A new millennial urologist must figure out how to incorporate new imaging modalities into their practice such as fusion biopsy, 7 T MRI, prostrate-specific membrane antigen, or PET-computed tomography. As novice physicians, they must train on newer technology such as single port robotics, high-intensity focused ultrasound, and radiofrequency ablation with few masters to guide them.[23] These millennials not only are interested in this technology, but they believe that technology will change the world.[24]

Millennials apply this new technology in ways that older generations may not be able to understand. They use the technology to make work more efficient. Their opinions should be a guiding force for developing strategy to gauge and change workplace trends. Based on behavior of millennials, practices can identify and gauge what needs to be changed. Based on millennial contributions, you can decide what needs to be brought forward and updated or discussed.[6]

As years passed, these technological advances began to come quicker and quicker. Starting with the Boomer generation, changes took off and within almost a decade, expectations quickly followed suit.[6] Now, the need and expectation for one to adapt and succeed almost instantly is a constant stress that millennials have to deal with. The unique ability of millennials to succeed and adapt to changes allows for appropriate adaptation in workforce technology progression as they train.

As these technological advances came, so did advances in knowledge. Knowledge is no longer limited, and the learning takes place at their fingertips.[25] Internet sites and databases are now available providing unique and specific medical knowledge to the training physician. The accessibility of these sites and this sort of knowledge to patients however provides a new avenue for a different kind of patient-provider relationship. Millennial physicians will need to work with some of the most well-informed patients and will need to include them and their thoughts in the care plan.[26]

## Key characteristics millennial urologist seek in practice

Millennial urologists want to be challenged, gain new knowledge and skills, and work in a positive environment.[8] Often as fresh medical school graduates or brand new attendings, millennial urologists are eager to use or explore the newfound set of skills and privileges that they have just been granted. In order to challenge this population, we must offer the opportunity for them to use those skills and the accompanying technology to solve how they can better treat the patients who need them.[23] As they recently stepped into a field of new and fresh technology and investigation, the ability and opportunity for these millennials to learn and hone these new skills is at the top of their list for criteria in a job. The advances in areas such as immunotherapy, genomics, microbiome, and transplantation all make urology an interesting avenue for millennials to gain this new knowledge and skill.[27]

### Work-life balance

A positive environment encompasses a positive work-life balance for a millennial physician. Millennials desire to work when they want and where they want. They hold the belief that time does not always equal productivity. Remember, they see fewer solid hours of work as more productive and beneficial than a day's worth of half-hearted work. They then hope to use this free time outside of work to spend it with their family or take up hobbies. Attractive positions to millennials involve not only the applicant but their families as well. Offering opportunities such as flexible scheduling or maternity and paternity policies will be more likely to draw a millennial physician just starting out with their new family. These millennials also expect a positive work environment. A toxic work culture has negative effects on employees and subsequently patients. Wellness initiatives should now be expected in physician training.[21]

### Potential of millennials

Recognizing the millennial physician and what makes them unique is the first step of having success with millennial physicians. The next step, however, would be to appreciate all that they have to offer. Growing up in a life of technology, they are not afraid of change and are always up for the task of learning new things. They embrace advances and are willing to apply what they know for the betterment of medicine. Their aptitude for technology and desire to grow allows for great contributions in urology. They are also more likely to take these skills and continue to improve via fellowship positions. Millennials in urology are more likely than previous generations to have completed a fellowship. For women and men under 45%, 62.5%, and 54.6% are fellowship trained, respectively. Compare this with 52.1% of women being fellowship trained and 29.4% of men being fellowship trained if they are older than 45 years.[1] With their less formal approach to relationships and mentoring, millennial physicians have the potential to break down barriers in the patient-provider relationship. Millennials are ambitious. They have grown up in families of helicopter parents who have told them they can do anything, and they believe it.

## SUMMARY

By recognizing, understanding, and appreciating the millennial physician, they can reach their potential. The proper encouragement and utilization of the millennial physician will create a loyal and driven workforce eager to grow and assist. Do not be discouraged by previous rumors of millennials as all coins have 2 sides. Listen to their requests in what they desire and be open to a different view of life than yours. A millennial's understanding of technology, grasp of patient-provider relationships, and desire to work hard may lead to the greatest generation of urologists.

## CLINICS CARE POINTS

- The millennial generation has experienced a unique upbringing providing them qualities to be successful physicians. Their familial, social, and educational background all mesh to form a caring, competent, and driven doctor.

- Media and older generations have often portrayed millennials in a negative light. It is key to not be discouraged by these opinions of millennials, as weaknesses are actually their greatest strengths.

- When adding a millennial urologist to your practice, you must remember what they have to offer and how you can appeal to their likings. Their family focus requires adequate work-life balance, sufficient benefits, and opportunity for growth.

- Fostered from a young age to take on challenges and roles that will provide success, a millennial will expect challenges that can push them in their career, technology to advance patient care, and mentorship to guide them along the correct paths.

# REFERENCES

1. American Urological Association. The State of Urology Workforce and Practice in the United States 2018. Linthicum, Maryland, April 5, 2019.
2. Duffin E. U.S. population by generation 2019. Statista. 2020. Available at: https://www.statista.com/statistics/797321/us-population-by-generation/. Accessed August 29, 2020.
3. What Does the American Dream Mean to Different Generations? Investopedia. 2019. Available at: https://www.investopedia.com/ask/answers/062215/what-does-american-dream-mean-different-generations.asp. Accessed February 22, 2020.
4. Weithing H, Sabadish N, Shierholz H. The class of 2012. Washington, DC: Economic Policy Institute; 2012. Available at: https://www.epi.org/publication/bp340-labor-market-young-graduates/. Accessed February 22, 2020.
5. Rich R. The great recession. Federal reserve history. 2013. Available at: https://www.federalreservehistory.org/essays/great_recession_of_200709. Accessed February 22, 2020.
6. Kadakia C. The millennial myth: transforming misunderstanding into workplace breakthroughs. Oakland (CA): Berrett-Koehler Publishers; 2017.
7. Martin K. Medscape residents salary & debt report 2020. New York: Medscape; 2019. Available at: https://www.medscape.com/slideshow/2019-residents-salary-debt-report-6011735#12. Accessed August 29, 2020.
8. Raines C. Connecting generations the sourcebook for a new workplace. Menlo Park (CA): Crisp Publications; 2003.
9. Dimock M. Defining generations: where millennials end and generation Z begins. Washington, DC: Pew Research Center; 2019. Available at: https://www.pewresearch.org/fact-tank/2019/01/17/where-millennials-end-and-generation-z-begins/. Accessed February 22, 2020.
10. Eckelberry-Hunt J, Tucciarone J. The challenges and opportunities of teaching "generation Y". J Grad Med Educ 2011;11(4):458–61.
11. Vanderveen K, Bold R. Effect of generational composition on the surgical workforce. Arch Surg 2008;143(3):224–6.
12. Guze P. Using technology to meet the challenges of medical education. Trans Am Clin Climatol Assoc 2015;126:260–70.
13. Borges N, Manuel RS, Elam C, et al. Differences in motives between Millennial and Generation X medical students. Med Educ 2010;44(5):570–6.
14. Burgess A, Bleasel J, Haq I, et al. Team-based learning (TBL) in the medical curriculum: better than PBL? BMC Med Educ 2017;17(1):243.
15. Teamwork: The Heart of Health Care. AAMC.org. 2016. Available at: https://www.aamc.org/news-insights/teamwork-heart-health-care. Accessed February 22, 2020.
16. Ende J. Feedback in clinical medical education. JAMA 1983;250(6):777–81.
17. Wljee J, Chopra V, Saint S. Mentoring Millennials. JAMA 2018;219(15):1547–8.
18. Hopkins L, Hampton B, Abbott J, et al. To the point: medical education, technology, and the millennial learner. Am J Obstet Gynecol 2018;218(2):188–92.
19. Han J, Rabley A, Vlasak A, et al. Career expectations and preferences of urology residency applicants. Urology 2019;123:44–52.
20. Kane L. Medscape National Physician Burnout & Suicide Report 2020: The Generational Divide. 2020. Available at: https://www.medscape.com/slideshow/2020-lifestyle-burnout-6012460. Accessed January 16, 2020.
21. Sharp M, Burkart K. Trainee wellness: why it matters and how to promote it. Ann Am Thorac Soc 2017;14(4):505–12.
22. Dell and intel future workforce study provides key insights into technology trends shaping the modern global workplace. San Francisco: Businesswire; 2016. Available at: https://www.businesswire.com/news/home/20160718005871/en/Dell-Intel-Future-Workforce-Study-Key-Insights. Accessed January 5, 2020.
23. Bernstein D, Bernstein B. Urological technology: where will we be in 20 years' time? Ther Adv Urol 2018;10(8):235–42.
24. Nieminen R. Information overload: strategies for achieving balance in a digital world. Interiors and sources. 2017. Available at: https://www.interiorsandsources.com/article-details/articleid/21738/title/information-overload-strategies-for-achieving-balance-in-a-digital-world/viewall/true. Accessed January 5, 2020.
25. Top apps for urologists. Urology Times 2016. Available at: https://www.urologytimes.com/view/top-apps-urologists. Accessed February 22, 2020.
26. Siwicki B. Apps for evidence-based medicine help physicians engage patients in shared decision-making. Healthcare IT News 2017. Available at: https://www.healthcareitnews.com/news/apps-evidence-based-medicine-help-physicians-engage-patients-shared-decision-making. Accessed December 29, 2019.
27. Key Advances in urology. Nature reviews urology. 2020. Available at: https://www.nature.com/collections/svfzkdtgxr. Accessed February 22, 2020.

# The Role of Advanced Practice Providers in Urology

Deepak A. Kapoor, MD*

## KEYWORDS

• Advanced practice providers • Nurse practitioners • Physician assistant

## KEY POINTS

- Population growth, particularly in the Medicare population, has greatly increased the need for urologic care in the United States—these needs cannot be met by urology as a specialty.
- Advanced practice providers (APPs) are unique providers of health care services who are practicing at the highest level of their certification and should be identified as such.
- Licensure and scope of practice requirements for nurse practitioners and physician assistants are governed at the state level and vary greatly by location.
- Billing regulations for practices that utilize APPs are complex; these must be understood and scrupulously followed.
- It is incumbent on urology as a specialty to recognize and address potential deficits in care and develop mechanisms to properly utilize APP resources to address these deficits.

## INTRODUCTION

The undersupply of urologists relative to need for urologic was anticipated in literature from early in the last decade.[1] More recently, the American Urological Association (AUA) annual census[2] identified 13,044 "practicing urologists" in the United States in 2019, an increase of 384 over the 12,660 reported in the 2018 report.[3] Of note, 85.6% (11,167) and 84.5% (10,693) were identified as active practicing urologists in 2019 and 2018, respectively. Consequently, the AUA census report suggests that the per capita ratio of urologists to the general population has improved from 3.72 to 3.99 urologists per 100,000 population in 2015 and 2019, respectively. Despite this increase, 62.4% of counties in the United States had no urologists in 2019.

Although on the surface, the AUA census data may provide some reassurance that the tide on urology manpower issues is beginning to be turned, this does not capture the extent of the problem, because the expansion of the Medicare population has exacerbated the shortage of urologists in the United States. The baby boom generation (born between 1946 and 1964) began to age into Medicare in 2011, when those born in 1946 turned age 65. This resulted in an immediate and dramatic increase in Medicare enrollment—daily Medicare enrollment increased by 16.6% in 2011 compared with 2010 (**Fig. 1**).[4] This trend has continued; since 2011, average new daily Medicare enrollment has increased by 21.4% compared with the 3 prior years. Even given disenrollment due to death and other causes, from 2008 to 2019, the Medicare rolls grew by more than 16 million beneficiaries, an increase of more than 29%.

Given the impact of Medicare expansion, a more appropriate analysis than total urologists per capita may be the number of urologists who treat Medicare beneficiaries, because this number is substantially lower than the number of urologists reported to be in active practice in the AUA census. As illustrated in **Fig. 2**, Medicare data

The Icahn School of Medicine at Mount Sinai, New York, NY, USA
* 340 Broadhollow Road, Farmingdale, NY 11735.
*E-mail address:* dkapoor@imppllc.com

Urol Clin N Am 48 (2021) 203–213
https://doi.org/10.1016/j.ucl.2021.02.001
0094-0143/21/© 2021 Elsevier Inc. All rights reserved.

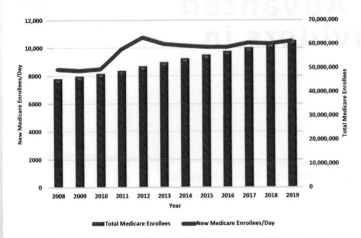

**Fig. 1.** New Medicare enrollees per day and total Medicare enrollees, 2008 to 2019.

suggest that the number of urologists that billed Medicare for any service from 2012 to 2018 increased by just over 0.5%, from 8792 to 8838, respectively.[5] Given the increase in Medicare beneficiaries, the per capita number of urologists was 17.3 to 14.7 per 100,000 Medicare beneficiaries in 2012 and 2018, respectively, a decrease in 14.9%. As illustrated in **Table 1**, when comparing the overall number of urologists, access for Medicare beneficiaries is worse; in 2018, 67.6% of the nation's 3144 counties had no urologists providing Medicare services compared with 62.4% of counties with no urologists at all ($P<.01$).[6] This is ominous particularly when considering that outcomes for the 3 most common genitourinary cancers is significantly worse in counties without urologic care.[7]

This article focuses on the role that advanced practice providers (APPs) can play to supplement the nation's urologic resources to expand access to services in a cost-effective manner.

## HISTORY AND TYPES OF ADVANCED PRACTICE PROVIDERS

Historically, APPs were characterized by the terms, *physician extenders* and *midlevel providers*. These terms should be discarded for several reasons. First, and most importantly, these terms are inaccurate—attempts to define individuals in these professions using these criteria tend to emphasize their role as appurtenant to a physician rather than as unique providers of service who are practicing at the highest level of their certification. As an extension, these definitions focus on what these professionals cannot or should not do rather than what they can do as part of their appropriate scope of practice. Second, these terms are inconsistent with the collaborative team approach to health care that is necessary to improve access, enhance outcomes, and reduce cost. Third, these historical definitions detract from the training and certification required to

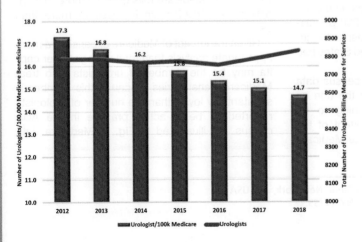

**Fig. 2.** Number of urologists billing for Medicare services and urologists/ 100,000 Medicare beneficiaries, 2012 to 2018.

**Table 1**
**Number of urologists per United States county, all urologists, and urologists billing Medicare**

| Number of Urologists in County | All Urologists, N (%) | Urologists Billing Medicare, N (%) |
|---|---|---|
| 0 | 1961 (62.4) | 2125 (67.6) |
| 1 | 294 (9.4) | 270 (8.6) |
| 2–3 | 299 (9.5) | 273 (8.7) |
| 4–8 | 263 (8.4) | 243 (7.7) |
| 9 or more | 327 (10.4) | 233 (7.4) |
| Total | 3144 (100.0) | 3144 (100.0) |

enter these professions, and many nurse practitioners (NPs) and physician assistants (PAs) find their use demeaning.[8]

Unquestionably, the earliest APPs were midwives; descriptions of midwifery as an independent profession date back millennium.[9] More recently, individuals without what would be considered formal medical education at the time continued to engage in the diagnosis and treatment of disease, both with and without formal physician supervision.[10] In the modern era, although any number of different professions can be considered APPs, this article focuses on NPs and PAs, because these are the predominant APPs involved in urologic care in the United States. The first formal training programs for both NPs and PAs were introduced in 1965, when Dr Loretta Ford and Dr Henry Silver developed the NP program at the University of Colorado and Dr Eugene A. Stead Jr created the first physician PA class at Duke University Medical Center. Over the subsequent years, the training and certification requirements for these fields have become codified. Although both serve important roles, there are important differences in training and scope of service between these professions.

To become a PA in the United States, it is necessary to be a graduate of an accredited PA program; as of January 2021, there were 315 such programs nationwide.[11] In general, these programs require 2 years to 3 years of study and usually result in a master of science (MS) degree. Certification requires evidence of degree status and between 1000 hours and 2000 hours of clinical practice as well as passing the Physician Assistant National Certifying Exam. Certification is required for licensure in all 50 states. Once certified, PAs use the designations, *PA-C* or *RPA-C*, where *C* connotes certified, and *R* is registered. These designations vary by state. More recently, doctoral programs for PAs that result in a doctor of medical science (DMSc) degree are being offered, but this degree is not required for practice.

There are a variety of NP designations, all categorized under the broad definition of advanced practice registered nurse (APRN). It is a prerequisite of APRN training to be a registered nurse, with subsequent 18 months to 36 months of post-baccalaureate training. It is not necessary to have clinical nursing experience to pursue APRN training. Although there are many types of APRNs, there are 4 broad categories of practice: (1) certified NP; (2) certified nurse midwife; (3) clinical nurse specialist; and (4) certified registered nurse anesthetist. Importantly, APRNs cannot be licensed only in a specialty area. Degrees commonly associated with APRNs are MS, MS in nursing, and doctor of nursing practice (DNP). Certification requires evidence of degree status as well as 500 hours to 1000 hours of clinical practice. As with the DMSc for PAs, the DNP degree is not required to practice.

## SCOPE OF PRACTICE

Scope of practice for both PAs and NPs varies according to state of practice and is a source of both confusion and controversy. In general, professional medical societies (led by the American Medical Association) contend that expansions of scope of practice will result in danger to patients due to the different levels of training of physicians and APPs.[12,13] As expected, societies representing APPs (American Academy of Physician Assistants and American Association of Nurse Practitioners) contend that expanding scope of practice for APPs will result in greater access, improve outcomes, and reduce costs—the global public health emergency (PHE) has provided momentum to these efforts.[14] Although exploration of this controversy is beyond the scope of this article, as with most circumstances with starkly opposing views from highly invested stakeholders, the truth likely is in the middle. Recent literature suggests that for most routine health care encounters, there is little evidence that quality of care rendered by APPs differs from physicians; simultaneously, diagnosis and management of more complex illnesses or patients with comorbidities are enhanced by physician supervision of care.[15]

For PAs, scope of practice laws are less complex than for NPs, because, by definition, PAs must function under the supervision of a physician. Scope of practice laws for PAs largely govern the mechanism by which physician supervision is provided as well as prescriptive authority for medications. At present, 47 states allow the supervising/collaborating physician at the practice site, 2 require a signed collaborative agreement between the PA and supervising physician, and 1 requires PAs to be directly supervised by a participating physician.[16] As with supervision requirements, prescribing rights in most states (44) is left to the discretion of the supervising physician, with only 6 states restricting the ability for PAs to prescribe Schedule II medication.[17]

For NPs, scope of practice is determined by the state in which the professional is licensed. There are 3 general categories that define scope of practice:

Full practice: state practice and licensure laws permit all NPs to evaluate patients; diagnose, order, and interpret diagnostic tests; and initiate and manage treatments, including prescribing medications and controlled substances, under the exclusive licensure authority of the state board of nursing.

Reduced practice: state practice and licensure laws reduce the ability of NPs to engage in at least 1 element of NP practice and require a signed collaborative agreement with a physician for the NP to provide patient care, or it limits the setting of 1 or more elements of NP practice.

Restricted practice: state requires supervision, delegation, or team management of NPs by physicians.

As of January 2021, 26 states or territories allow NPs full practice authority and 19 allow for reduced practice, whereas 11 restrict practice.[18]

An important exception to scope of practice regulations is for government employees. APPs employed by the federal government are not under jurisdiction of state scope of practice regulations, except with respect to the ability to prescribe and administer controlled substances. Importantly, in 2016 the US Department of Veterans Affairs (VA) amended provider regulations to permit full practice authority to 3 roles of VA APRNs to practice to the full extent of their education, training, and certification, regardless of state restrictions that limit such full practice authority, again, except for certain prescribing restrictions.[19]

Finally, during the PHE, waivers have been granted on the state level (which has jurisdiction over APP licensure) that ease supervisory requirements and scope of practice regulations for a variety of APPs. For PAs, 8 states have eased supervision requirements by executive order of their respective governor and 13 have suspended and/or waived all or partial supervision requirements by existing statute or regulation whereas 26 have suspended and/or waived select practice requirements (eg, licensure, ratios, and telemedicine)—only 3 states (Arkansas, Kentucky, and Alaska) have not taken waiver actions for PAs during the PHE.[20] NPs practicing in states or territories that do not permit full practice authority also have seen regulatory relief. Six states or territories have temporarily suspended all practice agreement requirements and 12 have issued temporary waiver of select practice agreement requirements, whereas 10 have taken no action on this issue.[21] In addition to state waivers, the federal government has issued several waivers to Medicare billing restrictions governing physician supervision at long term care facilities, provision of telemedicine, and the ability for hospitals to hire and utilize APPs to provide services.[22]

## BILLING CONSIDERATIONS FOR ADVANCED PRACTICE PROVIDERS

Historically, physicians have had disquiet about incorporating APPs into their practice due to concerns regarding financial liability. More recently, data suggest that in general, APPs can be incorporated into practices in a manner that is profitable,[23] with additional studies documenting this specifically for the specialty of urology.[24,25]

One issue that faces practitioners that incorporate APPs into their practice is the consideration of billing for services. Depending on the insurance company and the site of service, APPs may bill for services in 1 of 3 distinct methodologies: (1) incident-to billing, (2) direct billing, or (3) split/shared billing. The billing rules for each of these modalities are very specific, and although Medicare guidelines are national (albeit affected by state licensure rules), these rules may not apply to private payors. Further complicating the issue is that billing for APPs has been subject to an increase in the number of third party and Office of Inspector General (OIG) audits to ensure adherence to billing policies.

When permitted by scope of practice laws, APPs may bill carriers for their services directly. For Medicare, when this approach is utilized, the reimbursement is 85% of the rate listed in the Medicare Physician Fee Schedule. Private carriers each establish their own rate schedule for services directly billed by APPs, and although most follow Medicare policy, insurers are free to set fees that might be higher or lower than the percent used by Medicare. Although in some cases, fees paid to APPs may approach or equal physician fees, in no cases do they exceed physician payments. Other than overall reduced revenue from lesser reimbursement, there are 2 important considerations for when contemplating direct billing for APP services. The first is that if an APP is administering Part B drug payments, practices must ensure that these services are not subject to a contractual reduction in payment, because any such reductions may result in payments that are below acquisition costs. The second is that overhead costs for procedures, especially the costs of implants or disposables, must be factored when considering margins for procedures that are performed by an APP.

To avoid reimbursement and supervisory pitfalls, the most common approach to billing for APP services is "incident-to" billing. Services billed incident-to a physician service are reimbursed at 100% of the fee schedule for the physician provider. Although private payors can define this differently, the Medicare definition of incident-to billing covers services or supplies that are furnished as an integral, although incidental, part of the physician's personal professional services in the course of diagnosis or treatment of an injury or illness. These services are performed in the physician's office or in the patient's home and, during the PHE, may include telemedicine visits. Regulations vary by state regarding the scope and level of supervision required, but general requirements for the APP to qualify to bill for incident-to services include (1) a state license/registration; (2) a National Provider Identification (NPI) number; (3) being an employee of a physician or a physician-directed clinic as either a W-2 employee or a 1099 contracted/leased employee; (4) being under the control of the physician; and (5) presenting an expense to the physician, group practice, or legal entity. Qualifying incident-to service must be provided by a caregiver who is supervised directly, and, although private payors may have different payment rules, these services are reimbursed by Medicare at 100% of the applicable fee schedule.

An important caveat to billing for incident-to services is that the physician must perform the initial service, face to face with the patient, and document the plan of care which the APP will be following. As such, APP billing is incident-to the plan of care outlined by the physician billing provider at the initial visit with the patient. As such, 2 fundamental rules always must be observed for incident-to billing: (1) new patient visits performed by an APP are not considered incident-to physician services unless very strict documentation requirements are met, and any subsequent visits for the same diagnosis never can be billed as an incident-to visit; and (2) if an established patient being followed in accordance with incident-to regulations presents with a new problem, the APP may not bill as incident-to if the visit addresses the new problem, unless the physician documents participation in the visit and creates the new care plan. For example, a patient with advanced prostate cancer is placed on hormone deprivation therapy with an Luteinizing-hormone releasing hormone-antagonist, administered monthly by an APP. Administration of the medication and any services associated with the management of the advanced prostate cancer (as delineated in the physician care plan) are considered incident-to and may be billed at 100% of the applicable fee schedule. If, during a visit, however, the patients indicate another problem (such as urinary incontinence or erectile dysfunction), services referable to the new diagnosis may not be billed as incident-to unless the patient is evaluated for that specific issue by the physician and the physician issues a care plan for that problem.

There are additional provisions for APPs to bill for their services incident-to physician services. Although the billing physician does not have to be in the treatment room, he or she must be present within the suite of offices while the APP is performing the incident-to service. And although the billing provider does not have to be the physician who documented the plan of care, the billing/supervising provider must be present within the suite of offices and available to supervise/assist the APP who is performing the service. Importantly, the supervising physician cannot be performing a procedure while the incident-to services are being performed by the APP—in an audit, the OIG is looking to see where and what the supervising physician was doing at the time of the incident-to service; this information is readily available from the metadata incorporated into all certified electronic health records. As an aside, for multispecialty practices, the supervising physician does not have to be of the same specialty as the physician who performed the initial visit and created the patient plan of care. Finally, to qualify as an incident-to service, the APP must sign the medical record. Importantly, there is no incident-to billing in a hospital setting—these services must be billed under the APP as an independent service. Any services that are performed by APPs within a hospital setting are not paid if the licensing state and/or the insurance carrier does not allow for independent billing.

For split or shared billing, both the APP and the physician work for the same entity (ie, same practice or same hospital) and the service performed is an evaluation and management (E&M) service and not a consult or a procedure. The physician must provide the face-to-face portion of the E&M service with the patient (simply reviewing and agreeing with the APP's description on the patient's chart is not satisfactory to meet the requirement for split/shared billing). The APP and the physician see the patient on the same calendar day; if all criteria are met, then it is permissible to bill under the supervising physician's Medicare number, with payment at 100% of the fee schedule, but if not met, then the service must be bill under the APP's NPI with payment at 85% of the fee schedule. In split/shared visits, both the physician and the APP (PA or NP) must participate, each performing and documenting at least 1 required component of the E&M encounter. Split/shared visits may be performed for either initial or subsequent encounters at all levels of coding but not for consultative services, and this concept does not apply to critical care codes. It is important that each provider document their contribution to the service. Importantly, an addendum by the physician is not applicable; both physician and APP must contribute to the service being billed and the documentation must support distinct services for each provider. Again, if such an independent service is not permissible due to state regulations, then no payment for these services is made.

A final consideration when examining services performed by APPs are with respect to designated health services (DHSs). Payments for DHSs are subject to certain self-referral restrictions as delineated in federal Stark law. Guidelines regarding distribution of proceeds for DHSs performed by APPs billed by any of the methods described are arcane and complex—unfortunately, Stark law is a strict liability statute, and even unintentional technical violations can result in massive penalties. As such, practices must take great care that their income distribution formula with respect to DHSs performed by APPs is Stark compliant.

## SERVICES PERFORMED BY ADVANCED PRACTICE PROVIDERS

Over the past decade, both the number of APPs providing urologic services and the volume and nature of these services have increased. The 2019 AUA census reports that 71.4% of urologists incorporate APPs into their practice, an increase of 13.9% over the 2015 report.[2] Of the subset of urologists who utilize APP services, more than 79% interact with 2 or more APPs on a routine basis, suggesting that once the barrier to entry is overcome, physicians embrace the addition of APPs into their practice.

The most common services provided by APPs are E&M visits performed—due to the financial advantages, most of these are performed as incident-to visits. Depending on state of licensure and degree of training, however, APPs also may perform a variety of procedures as well as serve as surgical assistants. Because services performed by an APP incident-to a physician visit are billed under the physician's NPI number, ascertaining precisely how many procedures are performed by APPs is challenging. A review of service performed by APPs and directly billed, however, may provide insight into the general types of service performed. As illustrated in **Table 2**, a review of the Medicare billing data from 2012 to 2018 for Healthcare Common Procedural Coding System (HCPCS) codes referable to the most common urologic procedures (HCPCS 50000–55899) 20 HCPCS codes comprise nearly 99% of all APP direct billing for this period, with a single code (HCPCS code 51798, determination of postvoid residual urine) accounting for more than 55% of total services.[5]

As summarized in **Fig. 3**, the total number of APPs who directly billed for Medicare services increased from 1412 to 2557 in 2012 and 2018, respectively, an increase of 81.1%. Simultaneously, the total number of procedures directly billed to Medicare by APPs increased by 93.4%, from 186,673 in 2012 to 361,118 in 2018. During this interval, the ratio of urology procedures billed by APPs to Medicare compared with urology procedures billed by all providers to Medicare grew from 3.5% in 2012 to 6.8% in 2018, an increase of 95.7%.[5] The rate of expansion in number of services was significantly higher ($P = .04$) than the pace of expansion in the number of APPs providing these services, suggesting that these providers became progressively busier, particularly over the latter part of the last decade.[26]

Erickson and colleagues[27] found that most services provided by APPs could be considered an extension of routine urologic care. They concluded that these services, which can be learned relatively quickly but may be time consuming and disruptive to perform, could improve a practice's efficiency. At that time, more technical services (eg, cystourethroscopy, stent removal, and prostate biopsy) constituted a much smaller percent of APP direct

**Table 2**
Top 20 Healthcare Common Procedural Coding System codes direct billed to Medicare by advance practice providers by year

| Healthcare Common Procedural Coding System Code | Healthcare Common Procedural Coding System Description | 2012 (%) | 2013 (%) | 2014 (%) | 2015 (%) | 2016 (%) | 2017 (%) | 2018 (%) | Grand Total (%) |
|---|---|---|---|---|---|---|---|---|---|
| 51798 | Ultrasound measurement of bladder capacity after voiding | 56.4 | 51.9 | 52.3 | 54.8 | 55.7 | 56.4 | 56.3 | 55.1 |
| 51702 | Insertion of indwelling bladder catheter | 5.8 | 6.7 | 6.9 | 6.9 | 6.8 | 7.0 | 6.9 | 6.8 |
| 51701 | Insertion of temporary bladder catheter | 5.4 | 6.0 | 5.9 | 5.8 | 6.1 | 5.8 | 6. | 5.9 |
| 51741 | Complex uroflowmetry | 6.0 | 6.7 | 6.4 | 6.0 | 5.8 | 5.2 | 5.0 | 5.8 |
| 51700 | Bladder irrigation and/or instillation | 4.5 | 4.6 | 5.7 | 5.8 | 6.1 | 6.1 | 6.0 | 5.7 |
| 51720 | Bladder instillation of cancer preventive, inhibiting, or suppressive agent | 2.5 | 3.7 | 3.6 | 3.5 | 3.7 | 3.9 | 3.9 | 3.6 |
| 51784 | Non-needle measurement and recording of electrical activity of muscles at bladder and bowel openings | 5.2 | 5.5 | 4.2 | 3.1 | 2.7 | 2.6 | 2.4 | 3.4 |
| 51705 | Removal of skin suture with change of bladder tube | 2.0 | 2.7 | 3.2 | 3.0 | 3.4 | 3.5 | 3.9 | 3.2 |
| 51797 | Insertion of device into the abdomen with measurement of pressure and urine flow rate | 2.3 | 2.5 | 2.4 | 2.1 | 2.0 | 1.9 | 1.9 | 2.1 |
| 52000 | Diagnostic examination of the bladder and bladder canal (urethra) using an endoscope | 1.2 | 1.3 | 1.4 | 1.4 | 1.4 | 1.6 | 1.6 | 1.4 |

(continued on next page)

**Table 2** (*continued*)

| Healthcare Common Procedural Coding System Code | Healthcare Common Procedural Coding System Description | 2012 (%) | 2013 (%) | 2014 (%) | 2015 (%) | 2016 (%) | 2017 (%) | 2018 (%) | Grand Total (%) |
|---|---|---|---|---|---|---|---|---|---|
| 51728 | Insertion of electronic device into bladder with voiding pressure studies | 1.7 | 1.8 | 1.6 | 1.3 | 1.3 | 1.3 | 1.3 | 1.4 |
| 51729 | Insertion of electronic device into bladder with voiding and bladder canal (urethra) pressure studies | 1.0 | 1.1 | 1.1 | 0.9 | 0.8 | 0.8 | 0.8 | 0.9 |
| 55866 | Surgical removal of prostate and surrounding lymph nodes using an endoscope | 0.9 | 0.8 | 0.7 | 0.6 | 0.7 | 0.7 | 0.7 | 0.7 |
| 51703 | Insertion of indwelling bladder catheter | 0.4 | 0.6 | 0.9 | 0.9 | 0.8 | 0.7 | 0.6 | 0.7 |
| 53661 | Dilation of bladder canal (urethra), female | 0.8 | 0.8 | 0.7 | 0.6 | 0.3 | 0.2 | 0.2 | 0.4 |
| 51725 | Insertion of device into bladder to measure pressure of urine flow | 0.9 | 0.4 | 0.4 | 0.3 | 0.3 | 0.3 | 0.3 | 0.4 |
| 52310 | Removal of foreign body, stone, or stent from bladder canal (urethra) or bladder using an endoscope | 0.3 | 0.3 | 0.3 | 0.4 | 0.3 | 0.3 | 0.4 | 0.3 |
| 55700 | Biopsy of prostate gland | 0.5 | 0.4 | 0.4 | 0.4 | 0.3 | 0.3 | 0.2 | 0.3 |
| 54235 | Injection procedure to induce erection | 0.1 | 0.2 | 0.2 | 0.2 | 0.3 | 0.3 | 0.3 | 0.2 |
| 51792 | Assessment of muscle signal of pelvic nerves | 0.3 | 0.4 | 0.2% | 0.1 | 0.1 | 0.1 | 0.1 | 0.2 |

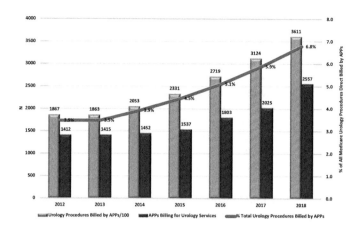

**Fig. 3.** Number of NPIs direct billing for Medicare services, total number of Medicare procedures/100 direct billed by APPs and percent of urologic and urologists/100,000 Medicare beneficiaries, 2012 to 2018.

billed services. Expanding the analysis, as described previously, suggests that although service volume expanded greatly, the nature of services provided did vary substantially; although there was a slight increase for both diagnostic cystourethroscopy and endoscopic stent removal (HCPCS codes 52000 and 52310, respectively), this was offset by a decrease in prostate biopsies (HCPCS code 55700) billed directly to Medicare by APPs.

## OPPORTUNITIES AND RISKS

The expanding shortage in access to urologic services provides ample opportunity for APPs to fill potential gaps in care. An immediate benefit to ramp up staffing on a national level is the duration of training required for an APP versus a physician to be able to practice to the full level of their certification; urologic education involves a minimum of 9 years of postgraduate education, not including fellowship, whereas an APP, can be licensed in approximately one-third that time. Increased staffing should enable faster patient access to care and potentially decrease burnout for overworked physicians (burnout has been identified as problematic particularly in the urologic community)[28]; burnout may be further reduced through enhanced after-hours on-call coverage. Because most services provided by APPs in an incident-to fashion involve managing cases according to a physician care plan as well as office procedures that should be mastered easily, physicians should be able to focus on more complex diagnostic, surgical, and patient management problems, improving quality of care and patient satisfaction. Clearly, practices that utilize APPs for other services, including office visits assisting in surgery, and seeing patients in a facility setting (eg, postoperative follow-ups, hospital consults, and emergency room visits) may

well experience lower operating overhead and other economic benefits by allowing physicians to continue to work in the more profitable office environment rather than spend time traveling between sites. Additionally, the advent of telemedicine services and the easing of billing and supervisory restrictions resulting from the PHE has opened additional opportunities to expand access to the many areas that either are without or are underserved from the perspective of urologic care. It remains to be seen if the temporary easing of restrictions will remain over the intermediate term to long term; if so, it can be anticipated that APPs will be an important component of care outreach to currently underserved communities. Finally, APPs are an opportunity for improve diversity in urologic caregivers. In its 2017 report on health care, 67.8 of PAs and 85.1% of APRNs were female[29]; contemporaneously, just 9.9% of the urologic workforce was female[2]; although this does not replace the need to encourage the development of female urologists, it will provide patients the opportunity to experience greater gender diversity in their contacts with urologic care. Regrettably, APPs do not provide a road to racial diversity; the same HHS report indicates that 84.0% of APRNs and 72.7% of PAs are white compared with 84.7% of practicing urologists[2,29]

Besides issues of regarding scope of practice and billing complexities identified previously, physicians grapple with issues of quality in APPs. Urologic training is not a core focus of training for APPs; as such, newly graduated APPs may need significant supervision and/or a specific urology training program prior to physicians having comfort in the care the APP may render. Although not linked directly to training, another issue of concern for supervising physicians is that of medical liability. Depending on the type of certification, APPs are between 12 times and 24 times less likely to be sued than physicians; that said, financial liability for claims still may be substantial.[30] In malpractice actions, the provider (physician or APP) may be held directly liable for their own acts or omissions, and the practice employing them may be subject to vicarious liability for failing to implement or enforce standard of care protocols. Liability actions involving APPs can be complicated by supervisory requirements, which may implicate the common law doctrine of *respondeat superior*, meaning "let the master answer." Using this doctrine, a physician can be held liable for liability claims occurring as a part of the APPs employment. This theory often is used to hold physicians liable for the acts or omissions of an APP. This situation can occur even when the physician did not treat the patient personally. Liability could arise because the physician employs the APP or because it is the physician's responsibility to supervise or oversee the APP. Because the definition of what constitutes appropriate collaboration or supervision of an APP varies greatly by type of PA and state of licensure, it is vital that physicians and practices familiarize themselves thoroughly with their then extant regulatory requirements regarding APP supervision.

## SUMMARY

Existing resources are inadequate to meet the nation's urologic health care needs. These access to care issues are exacerbated by the changing demographics of the population as well as the distributions of urologists nationwide; evidence suggests that this may be a greater problem for the Medicare population. Although utilization of APPs has increased recently, due to both an increase in number of caregivers and an apparent increase in services per APP, the nature of the services provided has not changed materially, focusing largely on E&M services and simple procedures. The shorter training period and demographics of the APP population have the potential to both address staffing issues and assist with gender diversity among urologic providers, but at least at present, increasing the number of APPs does not address racial diversity concerns. Expanding the role of APPs is complicated by the patchwork nature of licensure and supervision regulations that varies between states, payors, and type of APP. Practices that consider incorporating APPs must address issues of training, supervision, billing, and liability as well as ensuring compliance with Stark regulations should the APP perform DHSs. The current PHE has eased restrictions on APP services, loosened supervision requirements and expanded the availability of telehealth services—it remains to be seen if some or all these changes become permanent. Despite these challenges, APPs are an important resource whose role in providing urologic care is likely to continue to expand. As the principal caregivers of the genitourinary tract, it is imperative that the urologic community ensure the nation's access to urologic care, which includes actively engaging in ensuring quality of care by APPs by developing both training modules and possibly certification standards.

## DISCLOSURE

No disclosures.

## REFERENCES

1. Pruthi RS, Neuwahl S, Nielsen ME, et al. Recent trends in the urology workforce in the United States. Urology 2013 Nov 1;82(5):987–94.
2. American Urological Association. The State of Urology Workforce and Practice in the United States 2019. Available at: file:///C:/Users/dkapoor/AppData/Local/Temp/2019%20The%20State%20of%20the%20Urology%20Workforce%20Census%20Book.pdf.
3. American Urological Association, The State of Urology Workforce and Practice in the United States 2018. Available at: file:///C:/Users/dkapoor/AppData/Local/Temp/2018%20The%20State%20of%20the%20Urology%20Workforce%20Census%20Book-1.pdf.
4. Medicare Enrollment Dashboard. 2021. Available at: https://www.cms.gov/Research-Statistics-Data-and-Syste, ms/Statistics-Trends-and-Reports/CMSProgram Statistics/Dashboard.
5. Physician and Other Supplier Data CY 2012-2018. Available at: https://www.cms.gov/Research-Statistics-Data-and-Systems/Statistics-Trends-and-Reports/Medicare-Provider-Charge-Data/Physician-and-Other-Supplier.
6. Statistical analysis done with two-proportion z-test, performed using GraphPad Prism version 8.0.0 for Windows, GraphPad Software, San Diego (CA). Available at: www.graphpad.com.
7. Odisho AY, Cooperberg MR, Fradet V, et al. Urologist density and county-level urologic cancer mortality. J Clin Oncol 2010;28(15):2499.
8. Use of Terms Such as Mid-level Provider and Physician Extender: reviewed and revised by the AANP Fellows at the Winter 2015 Meeting. Available at: https://www.aanp.org/advocacy/advocacy-resource/position-statements/use-of-terms-such-as-mid-level-provider-and-physician-extender.
9. Bramall J, Towler J. Midwives in history and society. London: Croom Helm; 1986.

10. Keeling AW. Historical perspectives on an expanded role for nursing. Online J Issues Nurs 2015;20(2):2.

11. Physician Assistant Education Association: Our Programs. Available at: https://paeaonline.org/our-programs.

12. Robeznieks A. Why expanding APRN scope of practice is bad idea. Available at: https://www.ama-assn.org/practice-management/scope-practice/why-expanding-aprn-scope-practice-bad-ideaA.

13. Cabbabe S. Should nurse practitioners be allowed to practice independently? Mo Med 2016 Nov; 113(6):436.

14. Rosa WE, Fitzgerald M, Davis S, et al. Leveraging nurse practitioner capacities to achieve global health for all: COVID-19 and beyond. Int Nurs Rev 2020;67(4):554–9.

15. Sarzynski E, Barry H. Current evidence and controversies: Advanced practice providers in healthcare. Am J Manag Care 2019;25(8):366–8.

16. AMA Advocacy Resource Center. Physician assistant scope of practice. Available at: https://www.ama-assn.org/sites/ama-assn.org/files/corp/media-browser/public/arc-public/state-law-physician-assistant-scope-practice.pdf.

17. Scope of Practice Policy: Physician Assistants Overview. Available at: http://scopeofpracticepolicy.org/practitioners/physician-assistants/.

18. American Association of Nurse Practitioners, State Practice Environment. Available at: https://www.aanp.org/advocacy/state/state-practice-environment.

19. Advanced Practice Registered Nurses. 81 FR 90198 (December 16, 2016).

20. COVID-19 State Emergency Response, Suspended/Waived Practice Requirements. Available at: https://www.aapa.org/cme-central/national-health-priorities/covid-19-resource-center/covid-19-state-emergency-response/.

21. COVID-19 State Emergency Response: Temporarily Suspended and Waived Practice Agreement Requirements. Available at: https://www.aanp.org/advocacy/state/covid-19-state-emergency-response-temporarily-suspended-and-waived-practice-agreement-requirements.

22. Medicare and Medicaid Programs; Policy and Regulatory Revisions in Response to the COVID-19 Public Health Emergency. 85 FR 19230 (April 6, 2020).

23. Johnson JE, Garvin WS. Advanced practice nurses: Developing a business plan for an independent ambulatory clinical practice. Nurs Econ 2017; 35(3):126.

24. Swanton AR, Alzubaidi AN, Han Y, et al. Trends in operating room assistance for major urologic surgical procedures: an increasing role for advanced practice providers. Urology 2017;106:76–81.

25. Chen M, Kiechle J, Maher Z, et al. Use of advanced practice providers to improve patient access in urology. Urol Pract 2019;6(3):151–4.

26. Slopes of regression lines for number of APP NPIs billing Medicare and total procedures billed were compared with two-sample analysis of covariance (ANCOVA), performed using GraphPad Prism version 8.0.0 for Windows, GraphPad Software, San Diego (CA). Available at: www.graphpad.com.

27. Erickson BA, Han Y, Meeks W, et al. Increasing use of advanced practice providers for urological office procedural care in the United States. Urol Pract 2017;4(2):169–75.

28. Franc-Guimond J, McNeil B, Schlossberg SM, et al. Urologist burnout: Frequency, causes, and potential solutions to an unspoken entity. Can Urol Assoc J 2018;12(4):137.

29. Sex, race, and ethnic diversity of U.S. health occupations (2011-2015). U.S. Department of Health and Human Services, Health Resources and Services Administration; 2017. Available at: https://bhw.hrsa.gov/sites/default/files/bureau-health-workforce/data-research/diversity-us-health-occupations.pdf.

30. Hooker RS, Nicholson JG, Le T. Does the employment of physician assistants and nurse practitioners increase liability? J Med Regul 2009;95(2):6–16.

# Telemedicine in Urology
## The Socioeconomic Impact

Eric Kirshenbaum, MD[a],*, Eugene Y. Rhee, MD, MBA[b,c], Matthew Gettman, MD[d], Aaron Spitz, MD[e]

## KEYWORDS

- Telemedicine • Telehealth • Telesurgery • Urology • Disparities • Socioeconomic

## KEY POINTS

- The emergence of the COVID-19 public health emergency has propelled telemedicine into the future by alleviating many of the barriers that telehealth adopters faced.
- The Centers for Medicare & Medicaid Services have made several changes that allow practitioners to continue to utilize telemedicine through a variety of platforms.
- With the adoption of telemedicine came socioeconomic disparities in care and access. It is crucial to ensure equal access to this emerging technology.

## INTRODUCTION

In the year 2000, Reed Hastings, the founder and chief executive officer of a new start-up company based on movie rentals by mail, approached Blockbuster, a giant in the movie industry, to merge and lead Blockbuster's online brand. Blockbuster, rigid in its philosophy, refused to adapt with the online revolution and eventually filed for bankruptcy 10 years later. On the other hand, Reed Hastings grew his company to a current valuation of $125 billion and today Netflix leads the digital entertainment industry. This ability to adapt with changing times propelled Netflix into a leadership position in the industry. In many ways, telemedicine has the same trajectory as Netflix. An industry revolution for health care is transforming the ways in which health care is delivered. As usually happens, the adoption of disruptive technology varies greatly, and this may be exacerbated in certain socioeconomic demographics.

Although advocates of telemedicine have been frustrated by the historical lack of action in expanding telehealth services, the emergence of the COVID-19 public health emergency (PHE) virtually overnight has accelerated the adoption of telemedicine several years forward. This article reviews the recent changes in Centers for Medicare & Medicaid Services (CMS) rules regarding telemedicine and postulates its future impact; additionally, it focuses on the socioeconomic impact of telemedicine adoption on urology patients.

## BACKGROUND

Urologists will need to deliver telemedical care strategically in a scalable fashion that does not further the socioeconomic gap that already exists in health care. *Telemedicine* and *telehealth* are terms that describe the interactive exchange of health care information electronically between patients, providers, and consultants for the purpose of education, evaluation, decision making, and treatment. These interactions include text, audio, video, and audio-video communication. This may be live (synchronous) or as store-and-forward (asynchronous) interactions. Platforms are increasing and include personal computers, pads, tablets, smartphones, watches, wireless wearable sensors, and other emerging technologies. Under the official pronouncement by the federal government declaring COVID-19 a PHE,

[a] Uropartners, Suite 312, 1475 E Belvidere Rd, Grayslakle, IL 60030, USA; [b] Kaiser Permanente Urology, 4405 Vandever Ave, San Diego, CA 92120, USA; [c] Urology, Permanente Federation; [d] Mayo Clinic Department of Urology, 200 First Street SW, Rochester, MN 55905, USA; [e] Orange County Urology, 23961 Calle De La Magdalena, Laguna Hills, CA 92653, USA
* Corresponding author.
*E-mail address:* erickirs@gmail.com

Urol Clin N Am 48 (2021) 215–222
https://doi.org/10.1016/j.ucl.2021.01.006

waivers were issued that eased many telemedicine restrictions in a matter of weeks that had challenged the progress of telemedicine for years in the pre–COVID-19 era. Limitations on in-person visits due to safety concerns coupled with this liberalization of telemedicine requirements fast-tracked physicians across most specialties to integrate telemedicine into their practices. The early adoption of telemedicine by a minority of urologists helped onboard the vast majority of the nation's remaining urologists.

## WORKFORCE SHORTAGE

Telemedicine may provide a high-value solution for the workforce and access shortages in urology that have a disproportionate impact on communities from lower socioeconomic strata. The urology workforce will continue to be stressed with a progressive imbalance in available urologists to patients. It is estimated that by 2030, 20% of the population will be age 65 or older with increasing surgical needs. By 2030, urology will face a 32% (3884 urologists) shortage for greater than 350 million US citizens. According to the 2018 American Urological Association (AUA) census data, 30% of urologists are greater than 65 years old, a clear concerning sign of a progressive urologist shortage.[1] Urology is the second oldest specialty after thoracic surgery, confronting the profession with the prospect of losing a quarter of its workforce in a short period of time.[1,2]

Telemedicine can improve workforce efficiency and provide competitive advantages. Telemedicine can allow urologists to care for patients in larger geographic areas, addressing the scarcity of urologists in rural areas; 62.2% of US counties have 0 urologists, limiting patient access to necessary care. Even large urology groups may be challenged to meet the demands of their contracted population in urban and suburban markets but may use telemedicine to meet these challenges. Well after the COVID-19 PHE, telemedicine can allow urologists to leverage their subspecialty expertise across a larger population, allowing them to reach patients in need of their services whom they otherwise would not be able to encounter in person. Additionally, groups that adopt telemedicine for their patients' convenience will meet rising patient expectations for telemedical access, because many patients will have been introduced to telemedicine during the PHE who otherwise would not have. Traditional sectors of society already have incorporated and transformed a customer-centric focus, including travel, retail sales, and banking. Medicine will as well.

## PRE-COVID-19 TELEHEALTH COVERAGE

Prior to the PHE, health care reform, with its emphasis on value, was bringing more attention to the prospect of telemedicine. In many states, private payers were mandated to cover telemedicine services, often on par with office encounters. Medicaid covered telemedicine in almost all states. The Department of Veterans Affairs (VA) had been a true trailblazer in the world of telehealth. In 2019, the VA reported more than 900,000 veterans utilized its telehealth services (235% jump from previous year). Furthermore, the VA announced a 17% increase in televisits, delivering greater than 2.6 million telehealth episodes in 2019.[3]

Medicare had been very restrictive prior to the PHE, limiting coverage to remote geographies or certain chronic care scenarios but allowing some liberalization through alternative payment models, such as alternative care organizations or bundled payments. At the start of 2020, traditional Medicare and Medicare Advantage plans expanded telehealth coverage, limiting restrictions on patient location requirements and expanding coverage for more diagnosis.[4] As of March 1, 2020, during the PHE, traditional Medicare has radically liberalized access to telemedicine across effectively all locations and all conditions. The extent to which this will remain after the PHE has concluded is unknown, but even with a significant retraction, urologists can be well positioned to participate in alternative payment models that would compensate for telemedical services.

## TYPES OF TELEMEDICAL SERVICES
### Video Visits

A video visit is a live face-to-face electronic audio-video interaction between a provider and patient. Prior to the PHE, the combination of both audio and video was required by almost all payers for reimbursement. Telephone encounters are reimbursed by Medicare during the PHE but the extent to which that will remain is uncertain. Other payers may or may not provide reimbursement for telephone calls. In spite of the limitations of an on-screen encounter, video visits are successfully providing alternatives to traditional visits in a variety of settings, including clinic, office, urgent care, hospital, and skilled nursing facilities.

### Online Digital Evaluation Services

Patients may access portions of their electronic medical record and communicate with their urology care team. Value-added services also include online appointment scheduling, form submission such as history intake questionnaires, and online bill payment. Additionally, a practice can provide patient alerts for preventative services as well as definitions of conditions and guidelines and reminders for care, such as urology cancer rechecks. These services typically were not billable but they brought value to patients and helped satisfy government mandated meaningful use criteria for electronic health records.[5] During the PHE, traditional Medicare is reimbursing certain components of these services, known as virtual check-ins and digital evaluation services, whereby patients may communicate with their providers via text, e-mail, or chart portals, to determine the need for an in office visit or to efficiently address concerns not requiring an imminent office visit.

## eConsults

eConsults allow a urologist to asynchronously answer another provider's focused questions about the diagnosis or management of a specific patient. The urologist reviews the supporting material from the electronic medical record and provides a formal response to the focused question. Consultations most likely are solicited from large academic centers but also can be solicited from large urology groups. eConsults also can be synchronous (involving real-time interactions similar to video visits) and in this context also are known as video consults. In contrast to video visits, a patient typically is not present during a video consult. eConsults are performed using electronic software and hardware specifically for electronic consultations. For example, a portal called WebSphere (Cisco, San Jose, CA) has been used for eConsults. The response is documented in the medical record of the provider completing the eConsult.

eConsults are convenient for requesting providers and patients alike because they provide timely access to specialty expertise without requiring the patient to actually travel to visit with another urologist. Thus, eConsults allow patient visits to be completed in a shorter time frame and streamline the delivery of care. Scheduling also is more flexible with eConsults, especially asynchronous consults that can be completed outside of regular business hours. By using asynchronous eConsults particularly for more straightforward urologic problems, it is anticipated that more time would be spared for synchronous eConsults or traditional face-to-face consults on more complex patients during regular business hours. The concepts used in synchronous eConsults also have been applied to virtual tumor boards. Studies assessing the benefit of eConsults uniformly have demonstrated a reduction in the number of required in-person consults, ranging from 62% to 92%, optimizing patient time and physician efficiency.[6] With virtual tumor boards, detailed case presentations are made in the same way as traditional tumor boards. Radiologic studies and histologic findings are reviewed ahead of time with a radiologist and pathologist, respectively. Using this approach, a second opinion for the patient is obtained and the mechanism is a powerful means to keep high standards of clinical care and performance within the control of a private large group practice.

## Tele-intraoperative Consultation

Although adoption is still in its infancy, the intraoperative consultation is perhaps the most innovative and valuable application of telemedicine. The urologist offers electronic consultations regarding intraoperative findings with other surgeons remotely. Tele-intraoperative consultations promise to enhance productivity and surgical quality as this matures. Hung and colleagues[7] categorized currently available telesurgical technologies into 4 categories: verbal guidance, telestration, guidance with teleassist, and telesurgery. Verbal guidance is simply a 2-way communication between surgeon and consultant with video monitoring, the benefit being it is easily implemented with low cost and minimal bandwidth requirements. Telestration allows a consultant or mentor to telestrate in 2-dimensions or 3-dimensions, aiding the surgeon through various aspects of a procedure. TIMS Consultant (TIMS Medical, Chelmsford, Massachusetts), an interactive video broadcast network within hospitals, such as Kaiser Permanente, provides high-resolution, live video streams anywhere remotely, including compliant smartphones and laptop computers. Remote multiparty interactivity and collaboration are provided through integrated audio conferencing and live telestrations. Teleassists allow for the mentor or consultant to reach into the patient remotely and physically aid in a procedure. Lastly, telesurgery allows for the entire surgery to be completed remotely.[7] Sterbis and colleagues[8] performed 4 porcine radical nephrectomies utilizing the daVinci robot (Intuitive Surgical: Sunnyvale, CA) from greater than 1300 miles away.

## Telementoring and Teleproctoring

A urologist can serve as a mentor and/or proctor during a telesurgical procedure creating telementoring and teleproctoring services.[9–12] This has broad implications with licensure and credentialing in the practice of urology. Telementoring and teleproctoring can address cumbersome and impractical barriers posed by physical proctoring. Hinat and colleagues,[13] in 1 of the first reported series of telementoring and teleproctoring in robotics, used a telementoring system to promote surgical techniques associated with robotic-assisted radical prostatectomies. The group demonstrated proper function and acceptable latency with no differences in surgical outcomes, incline operative times, complication rates, early continence status, and positive margin rates between the telementoring and direct mentoring groups.

### Telesimulation and Telesurgical Rehearsal

Simulators now are being used to teach minimally invasive surgical techniques. A network of simulators can assist teaching and evaluating novice surgeons and those who desire improvement. Simulators can standardize teaching and as well allow for interactive proctoring during the simulated procedures. A surgical dress rehearsal may be possible before the actual operation. Currently, urology patient–specific simulations are in development that could be integrated into established training programs rapidly and easily.

### Telemedicine: Systems and Procedures

As with traditional care delivery, telemedicine can be enhanced by following standard operating procedures. General and specialty medical societies currently are generating guidelines for telemedicine that include technical instructions and ethical considerations. Guidelines also increase the delivery of high-quality and safe patient care, key themes needed for telemedicine to be supported by legislators and payers.

Prior to the PHE, telemedicine was required to be delivered using secure Internet-based videoconferencing technologies. During the PHE, encrypted platforms still are encouraged but not required by Medicare when their unavailability creates a barrier to access. Non–Health Insurance Portability and Accountability Act (HIPAA) compliant platforms, such as FaceTime, are allowable but public facing platforms, such as Facebook Live, are not. Furthermore, during the PHE, telephone encounters may be conducted for reimbursement on par with video encounters. Nonetheless, after the PHE, telephone-only encounters may or may not continue to be reimbursed and HIPAA requirements for secure connections likely will return. It is advisable to select a secure video platform for a long-term telemedical strategy. The network used for telemedicine typically is a secure virtual private network,

with software that typically is licensed to a host institution. Videoconferencing with encryption software can be downloaded to connect with patients directly in their own homes or other noninstitutional settings. Internet-based platforms also can be used as an alternative portal for urologists and patients seeking telemedicine services. Telemedical encounters also may be initiated by patients via direct-to-consumer telemedical companies, such as Hims and Roman, which specialize in select male health concerns.

For practices considering implementation of video visits, it is useful to consider the urologic diagnoses for which video visits will be most effective. The experience with many urologists during the PHE is that most, if not all, diagnoses can be managed in part or in whole with telemedicine. Telemedicine need not be an either/or proposition, such that a visit that is conducted telemedically does not preclude a prompt follow-up in-person visit when deemed necessary.

Informed consent is established prior to the start of the video visit. The consent typically is conducted in real time following laws within a patient's jurisdiction. The provider should document the consent in the medical record. The consent should include a discussion about the structure and timing of services, record keeping, scheduling, privacy, risks, confidentiality, mandatory reporting, and billing. Confidentiality and the limits of confidentiality in electronic communication also should be discussed. It also is important that the issue of video recordings be discussed. Specifics regarding technical failure of the video visit, protocols for contact between sessions, and conditions upon which the video visits will be terminated in lieu of a traditional visit also need to be established.

Video visits need to be carried out in an appropriate environment for both the provider and the patient to maximize privacy. Video cameras and lighting should be optimized for both the patient and provider during a video visit. If a patient attempts to carry out a video visit in a public space, the provider should recommend that the consultation be delayed until a suitable private space is identified. The consultation should start with identity verification of both the provider and patient. In many instances, a host clinic may perform the verification prior to starting the video visit. The location of the provider and the patient also should be established during the video visit. Contact information for both the provider and the patient should be verified during the video visit. Lastly, the expectations regarding the video visit and any subsequent visits should be discussed.

The urologist must make an entry in the medical record in a fashion similar to that for traditional visits once the video visit is complete. The medical record entry should include an assessment and plan, patient information, contact information, history, informed consent, and information regarding fees and billing. As part of the documentation, it also is important to note that the patient was seen using telemedicine technologies.

Regarding connectivity, audio-video telemedicine services can be provided through personal computers or mobile devices that use Internet-based videoconferencing software programs. A bandwidth of 384 kilobits per second or higher in both the downlink and uplink directions is recommended.[2] Because different technologies provide different video quality results at the same bandwidth, each endpoint should use a bandwidth sufficient to achieve at least a minimum of 640 pixels × 360 pixels resolution at 30 frames per second. Each party should use the most reliable connection to the Internet during the video visit.

Next, it is important to verify the patient has the required hardware and software capabilities for a video visit and sufficient broadband connectivity. The patient should be provided contact information for technical support in case troubleshooting is required. Rather than have the patient manage the requirements of the video visit, another option is for the patient to report to a telemedicine center where the hardware, software, and connectivity are provided and standardized for maximum reliability.

The increasing availability of 5G networks throughout the country will have a significant impact on telehealth availability as adequate information technology infrastructure will be available to remote patients and clinicians; 5G wireless ecosystems will continue to grow, given both regional and national initiatives from network and wireless providers. Compared with 4G, 5G can be expected to be 100-times faster, with 25-times lower lag times and 1 million devices supported in 1 square mile. The 5G systems will allow for reliable, faster connections, resulting in high-quality video connections and data transfer.[14]

Efforts should be taken to make audio and video transmission secure by using point-to-point encryption that meets recognized standards. Currently, Federal Information Processing Standard Publication 140-2, is the US Government security standard used to accredit software encryption and lists encryption types, such as advanced encryption standard, as providing acceptable levels of security. When patients or providers use a mobile device, special attention should be paid to the relative privacy of information being communicated over such technology. Mobile devices should require a passcode and should be configured to have an inactivity timeout function not exceeding 15 minutes.

## GAPS TO ACCESS

With the emergence of telemedicine in urology came socioeconomic inequalities in care. Many patients do not possess the basic technology required for a robust telehealth visit. In the initial PHE rules, telephone encounters were not included creating an access gap for those who did not have adequate Internet, smartphones, or computers. On March 31, 2020, CMS allowed for telephone services to be covered during the PHE (Current Procedural Terminology code 99441-99443), including creating parity between telephone and televideo visits. This bridged a significant access gap for those unable to perform video visits.

Prior to the PHE, coverage and reimbursement for telephone calls were severely limited. G2021 Healthcare Common Procedure Coding System (HCPCS) code (brief communication technology-based service) seldom was used and had limited reimbursement. Although telephone coverage expanded access, investigators are assessing its adequacy as a telemedical platform. The utilization of telephone calls was studied by Safir and colleagues,[15] who compared telephone with face-to-face encounters for hematuria consults in the VA population. They found access improved from 72 days to 12 days, although overall satisfaction with visit was higher in the face-to-face visit cohort (92% VS 84%).

The launch of telemedicine in the Bronx, New York during the PHE offers a glimpse into its utilization and limits in a socioeconomically disadvantaged population. Montefiore Medical Center, one of the largest and diverse hospital systems in the country, transitioned almost overnight to 95% telehealth visits. This was in a population where approximately 50% of households did not have adequate Internet access, 20% preferred non-English language, 44% relied on Medicaid, and 40% lived in poverty. The group found 88% satisfaction with video visits and 81% for telephone-only encounters; 67% of patients felt they received similar care as in office visit whereas 79% would choose a telemedicine encounter. Similar to previous research, clear travel time and clinic wait time advantages were seen for telehealth. Lastly, there was a preference for phone visits compared with video visits, a majority citing technologic limitations as the reason telephone is preferred.[16] This small study highlights the need for continued expansion of telephone-only encounters.

Although CMS has recognized telephone services as telehealth by adding them to Medicare telehealth services, the degree of coverage beyond the PHE has yet to be seen. CMS understood the importance of this technology because it allowed for social distancing and expanded access for underserved populations. As the new 2021 CMS rule currently stands, telephone-only encounters will not continue after the PHE. CMS, however, did introduce G2252 HCPCS code, which is a virtual check-in for established patients with incremental times to account for differing time spent on the phone. This will lead to a significant cut in relative value unit per time spent with patients on phone. In addition, this cannot lead to an in-person visit within 7 days and may not result from a recent visit.

## NEW 2021 CENTERS FOR MEDICARE & MEDICAID SERVICES RULES

Several changes in the 2021 CMS rules will have a long-lasting impact on providers and patients utilizing telemedicine. The most significant change in the 2021 rules is the emphasis on medical decision making (MDM) when determining levels of service. No longer are particular history and physical examination components required; rather, providers determine level of service on MDM alone. The history and examination are left to the discretion of the provider to perform what is medically appropriate. By eliminating the physical examination requirements, providers can focus on MDM and be reimbursed for their work based on the complexity of the patient. This is important especially when utilizing telemedicine because the ability to perform a comprehensive physical examination is limited. By way of example, a new patient with metastatic prostate cancer with multiple complicating factors can be billed at the same level as an in-person encounter because CMS no longer requires the detailed physical examination previously required. Furthermore, for time-based billing, the total time now includes previsit and postvisit preparation and coordination. For many providers, this better represents the amount of time it takes to care of patients. Although the telehealth visit itself may take only 10 minutes, CMS now reimburses for time spent reviewing imaging, records, and coordinating care at the conclusion of the visit.

### Evaluation and Management Changes

During the PHE, the list of covered telehealth services was expanded significantly. Some of these

**Table 1**
**Current procedural terminology codes for services covered through 2021**

| | |
|---|---|
| Rest home visits | 99336-99337 |
| Home visits | 99349-99350 |
| Therapy services | 97161-97168, 97110, 97112, 97116, 97535, 97750, 97755, 97760, 97761, 92521-92524, 92507 |
| Critical care codes | 99469, 99472, 99476, 99478-99480, 99291-99292 |
| Discharge codes | 99315-99316, 99238-99239, |
| Observation management | 99217, 99224-99226 |
| Emergency department | 99281-99285 |

are set to expire after the PHE whereas others were added to the permanent covered services. A list of services covered through 2021 is in **Table 1**.

For the time being, many of the restrictions associated with originating sites will revert back to pre-PHE rules when the PHE expires. This means that services covered on the PHE list, including evaluation and management codes, will be restricted to those in rural areas (health shortage regions) and at approved facilities. Legislation surrounding the originating site is expected to change because there is a strong push to permanently eliminate originating site restrictions. One area of particular interest is the status of remote patient monitoring and its reimbursement. This has the potential to expand the diagnostic reach to patients in more rural areas of the country bridging significant geographic disparities in care. The final rule states that remote patient monitoring can be used for established patients but must be a Food and Drug Administration–approved device with certain data collection requirements.

### Advanced Practice Providers

The role for advanced practice providers (APPs) has expanded exponentially over the past decade. There is a projected shortage of physicians, ranging from 46,000 to 121,000 by 2032. Urology is likely to be plagued greatly by this shortage given it is the second oldest surgical specialty, with more than 18% of its workforce greater than 65 years old.[2] Although increasing the role of APPs potentially can address this workforce shortage, adequate supervision is imperative. Technology-based supervision has the potential to expand access with an increasing APP workforce while simultaneously providing adequate and efficient supervision. During the PHE, CMS has allowed for supervision of APPs utilizing audio and visual technology. There are new CMS rules surrounding direct supervision of APPs. Direct supervision traditionally meant that a physician must be in the same office and immediately available to assist. During the PHE, direct supervision is able to be accomplished through combined audio-video communication. Audio alone does not satisfy the requirement. This allows APPs to perform procedures and see patients without the overseeing doctor being physically in the office. This has been extended until December 31, 2021, or the end of the PHE, whichever is later.

## DISPARITY IN TELEMEDICINE CARE

With the accelerated rise in telehealth adoption, many healthcare professionals are concerned that this has resulted in an unequal distribution of health care resources, further widening racial and socioeconomic disparities. At its inception, telemedicine was meant to expand the health care reach to underserved populations and those living in rural areas. With telehealth companies focusing on well-resourced patients in order to expand their market presence, the concern is that those for whom telehealth initially was intended will be left behind. Furthermore, relying on telehealth algorithms for care risks magnifying disparities because underrepresented populations often are not included in algorithmic data. Few studies have assessed the socioeconomic impact of the rapid changes in telehealth that have occurred under the PHE. Weber and colleagues,[17] a group from one of the largest health care systems in New York City, evaluated telehealth utilization for COVID-19-related care at the height of the initial COVID-19 wave. They found that compared with whites, blacks and Hispanics were more likely to go in person to emergency rooms and in-office visits rather than utilizing telehealth services. Similarly, patients greater than 65 years old utilized in-person emergency room and office visits at higher rates than their younger cohort. Similarly, Eberly and colleagues[18] reviewed records of 150,000 patients who scheduled telemedicine visits at the beginning of the pandemic (March 2020–May 2020). They found that 54% of patients followed through with their visit. Furthermore, they found disparities in utilization for age, race, and income. They found that when comparing utilization of video visits versus telephone encounters there

was a lower video utilization in women, blacks, Hispanics, and low-income families.[17,18] Some reasons for this inequality include technology barriers for older patients, language barriers, Internet constraints in lower-income patients, and lack of adaptations for those with disabilities (ie, visually and hearing impaired). Because there may be benefits unique to video visits as providers are able to examine patients visually and pick up on various visual cues, it is important for physicians, hospitals, politicians, and insurers to ensure equal representation in all telehealth services.

## CONTEMPORARY (PUBLIC HEALTH EMERGENCY) UTILIZATION

The emergence of COVID-19 and the subsequent PHE propelled telemedicine into the future. Urologists were quick to adopt telemedicine to facilitate social distancing, continue care for their patients, and keep practices financially viable. Urology saw a dramatic acceleration of utilization, with 71.5% of urologists stating they participated in telemedicine during the PHE according to the 2020 AUA annual census data. The most common telemedicine topics were benign prostatic hyperplasia, elevated prostate-specific antigen, erectile dysfunction, stone disease, and voiding dysfunction. Approximately half of urologists provided telemedicine encounters for new patients and 77% provided encounters for established patients. According to census data, of those urologists participating in telemedicine, urologists receive compensation primarily for video visits (93.9%) and telephone calls (77%) whereas fewer than 11% reported receiving compensation for eConsults, video visits with other providers, and text messages.

## SUMMARY

Just as Reed Hastings adapted to the changing landscape of movie rentals, so has the field of urology adapted with the rapid emergence of telehealth. Telemedicine appears positioned to be a mainstay of health care systems beyond the PHE and urologists are well positioned to pioneer the expansion of services. In addition to meeting the current demands for social distancing arising from the pandemic, telemedicine specifically may help address the needs of underserved communities by addressing workforce shortages. It also will prove instrumental to increasing clinical and surgical productivity, improving patient access to care, and facilitating data quality reporting. It is crucial to focus on those who benefit most from this new technology (ie, underserved populations) and ensure equal access. As the initial limitations have been radically removed and as new solutions are developed both in the technology and regulatory sides, it is possible that telemedicine will become completely integrated into urologic training and health care delivery to fulfill its promise of access and quality urologic care.

## DISCLOSURE

The authors have nothing to disclose.

## REFERENCES

1. Jennifer M. Ortman and Christine E. Guarneri: United States population Projections: 2000 to 2050. United States Census Bureau; 2009. Available at: https://www.census.gov/content/dam/Census/library/working-papers/2009/demo/us-pop-proj-2000-2050/analytical-document09.pdf.
2. Nuewahl: AAMC projection through 2025. AAMC; 2012. Available at: https://www.aamc.org/media/45976/download.
3. Anon: VA reports significant increase in Veteran use of telehealth services. United States Department of Veterans Affairs; 2019. Available at: https://www.va.gov/opa/pressrel/pressrelease.cfm?id=5365#:~:text=WASHINGTON%20%E2%80%93%20The%20U.S.%20Department%20of,telehealth%20care%20in%20FY%202019.
4. Anon: Telehealth Coverage. Medicare.gov. Available at: https://www.medicare.gov/coverage/telehealth, Accessed January 21, 2020.
5. Anon: Website. Meaningful use definition & objectives. 2015. Available at: HealthIT.gov; HealthIT.gov https://www.healthit.gov/providers-professionals/meaningful-use-definition-objectives. Accessed September 13, 2016, Accessed January 21, 2021.
6. Modi PK, Portney D, Hollenbeck BK, et al. Engaging telehealth to drive value-based urology. Curr Opin Urol 2018;28:342–7.
7. Hung AJ, Chen J, Shah A, et al. Telementoring and Telesurgery for Minimally Invasive Procedures. J Urol 2018;199:355–69.
8. Sterbis JR, Hanly EJ, Herman BC, et al. Transcontinental Telesurgical Nephrectomy Using the da Vinci Robot in a Porcine Model. Urology 2008;71:971–3.
9. Sathiyakumar V, Apfeld JC, Obremskey WT, et al. Prospective randomized controlled trial using telemedicine for follow-ups in an orthopedic trauma population. J Orthop Trauma 2015;29:e139–45.
10. Hwa K, Wren SM. Telehealth follow-up in lieu of postoperative clinic visit for ambulatory surgery: results of a pilot program. JAMA Surg 2013;148:823–7.
11. Matimba A, Woodward R, Tambo E, et al. Teleophthalmology: Opportunities for improving diabetes eye care in resource- and specialist-limited Sub-Saharan African countries. J Telemed Telecare 2016;22:311–6.
12. Canon S, Shera A, Patel A, et al. A pilot study of telemedicine for post-operative urological care in children. J Telemed Telecare 2014;20:427–30.
13. Hinata N, Miyake H, Kurahashi T, et al. Novel telementoring system for robot-assisted radical prostatectomy: impact on the learning curve. Urology 2014;83:1088–92.
14. Editorial Team: 5G vs. 4G - A Side-by-Side Comparison. 2019. Available at: https://datamakespossible.westerndigital.com/5g-vs-4g-side-by-side-comparison/. Accessed January 21, 2021.
15. Safir IJ, Gabale S, David SA, et al. Implementation of a Tele-urology Program for Outpatient Hematuria Referrals: Initial Results and Patient Satisfaction. Urology 2016;97:33–9.
16. Watts KL, Abraham N. "Virtually perfect" for some but perhaps not for all: launching telemedicine in the bronx during the COVID-19 pandemic. J Urol 2020;204:903–4.
17. Weber E, Miller SJ, Astha V, et al. Characteristics of telehealth users in NYC for COVID-related care during the coronavirus pandemic. J Am Med Inform Assoc 2020;27:1949–54.
18. Eberly LA, Khatana SAM, Nathan AS, et al. Telemedicine outpatient cardiovascular care during the COVID-19 pandemic: bridging or opening the digital divide? Circulation 2020;142:510–2.

# The Growth of Integrated Care Models in Urology

Caitlin Shepherd, MD[a],*, Michael Cookson, MD[b], Neal Shore, MD[c]

## KEYWORDS

- Multidisciplinary communication • Integrated health care systems • Integrative oncology
- Value-based purchasing • Telehealth • Genitourinary cancers • Bladder cancer • Prostate cancer

## KEY POINTS

- Integrated health care models align health care providers and specialists to improve care coordination, diagnostic accuracy, shared decision making, and the delivery of timely, appropriate, evidence-based treatment, while ultimately reducing health care costs.
- For some urology practices and clinics, integrated health care models are an untapped resource that can improve patient outcomes and maintain reimbursements in the era of alternative payment models.
- Integrated care benefits all patients in urology, from pediatrics through transitional care and into adulthood.
- Multidisciplinary clinics (MDCs) are now the standard of care for managing genitourinary malignancies and show promise in other malignant and nonmalignant genitourinary diseases and conditions.
- Implementing MDCs can be resource-intensive and time-consuming, but in most settings, improved care coordination and treatment access ultimately reduces health care costs.

## INTRODUCTION

Integrated health care models are increasingly sought in modern medicine. With recent health care reforms and the preference for value-based over volume-based health care, there is ongoing interest and emphasis on population health and evidence-based care that correlates patient outcomes and pathways with reimbursement metrics. Organizations such as Geisinger, Kaiser Permanente, and the Department of Veterans Affairs are well-known examples of large, fully integrated health care systems that attempt to improve quality, efficiency, and patient outcomes.[1] The integrated health care model has permeated over the years into regional health care systems and community clinics.

## DEFINITIONS

Integrated health care models are organized, collaborative networks that aim to align health care providers who are clinically and/or fiscally accountable for patient populations across the care continuum.[2] The model should focus on a fully coordinated, evidence-based health care systems approach chiefly designed to manage and improve clinical outcomes.

## IMPORTANCE

As has been recognized, integrated care models are associated with enhanced health care utilization, cost efficiencies, and patient outcomes. This model of health care delivery represents an

[a] University of Oklahoma, 920 Stanton L. Young Boulevard, WP 2140, Oklahoma City, OK 73104, USA; [b] Department of Urology, University of Oklahoma, 920 Stanton L. Young Boulevard, WP 2140, Oklahoma City, OK, USA; [c] CPI, Carolina Research Center, 823 82nd Parkway, Myrtle Beach, SC 29572, USA
* Corresponding author.
*E-mail address:* Caitlin-Shepherd@ouhsc.edu

Urol Clin N Am 48 (2021) 223–232
https://doi.org/10.1016/j.ucl.2020.12.002

untapped resource for some urology practices and clinics and can potentially improve outcomes in general, reconstructive, and pediatric urology, as well as urologic oncology.[3]

Because urologic conditions are most prevalent among older individuals, urologists often manage patients with comorbidities who receive multiple medications or are subjected to polypharmacy and whose care involves several specialists. This can potentially fragment health care delivery, leading to preventable hospitalizations, suboptimal health care outcomes, decreased quality of life, and greater health care costs.[4] Integrating care can address these challenges and is vital for both younger and older urology patients.

## BRIEF HISTORY OF INTEGRATED HEALTH CARE

The evolution of integrated care in the United Started began as an attempt to manage escalating health care costs associated with fee-for-service payment structures that incentivized volume of care instead of quality of care. Under a traditional fee-for-service model, patients received inconsistent care due to a lack of standardization of practices and a disjointed physician landscape.[5] The goal of integrated (or accountable) care is to improve patient outcomes and experiences while reducing costs associated with a specific health care delivery.

Historically, attempts at health care reform led to mixed results from Health Maintenance Organizations in the 1980s and 1990s and the Medicare Physician Group Practice Demonstration in the early 2000s.[5] However, in 2008, Accountable Care Organizations (ACOs) were initiated to reform health care delivery by transitioning fee-for-service payment structures toward more accountable, value-based reimbursement. Physicians would therefore be motivated to provide health care more efficiently to not only lower costs but also increase quality. As part of the 2010 Patient Protection and Affordable Care Act, ACOs have become the leading alternative payment model to be used by the Centers for Medicare and Medicaid Services.[6] This model attempts to alter health care implementation toward a value-based model and is potentially very impactful for the practice of urology, which has a preponderance of patients receiving Medicare benefits.

However, a recent study showed that only 10% of practicing urologists participated in ACOs.[7] Contributing factors may include cumbersome regulatory burdens, the instruction required for implementation, and the fact that urology is a surgical subspecialty for which clear alternative payment models have not evolved. There is some trending toward an increased transition from volume-based to value-based models, but the complexities of the health care system and ongoing health policy debates continue to thwart the implementation of optimal integrated systems.

## VALUE OF MULTIDISCIPLINARY CARE IN ONCOLOGY

Multidisciplinary expertise is widely accepted as crucial for decision making in cancer care, particularly for complex clinical cases. Compared with health care facilities that lack an integrative care model, multidisciplinary clinics are more likely to follow evidence-based practice recommendations and are associated with fewer unnecessary delays between diagnosis and treatment, greater diagnostic accuracy guided by expert radiology and pathology review, and improved patient satisfaction scores. Multidisciplinary clinics have become common in the management of many types of non-genitourinary cancer, and their use has been shown to significantly alter patient management. Indeed, in published studies, multidisciplinary clinics changed case interpretation and/or treatment in 45% of patients with breast cancer, 23% of patients with myeloma, and 24% of patients with pancreatic cancer.[8–12]

## CURRENT INTEGRATED CARE MODELS IN UROLOGY

Integrated care positively impacts care for all patients. However, select populations in urology benefit most from this model of health care delivery. Examples include patients with complex pediatric genitourinary conditions, neuro-urologic disorders, interstitial cystitis or bladder pain syndrome, and complex urologic tumors. **Fig. 1** demonstrates an example of integrated health care in urology. We briefly discuss each of these populations and provide examples of how multidisciplinary clinics help streamline care and improve outcomes.

### Pediatric Urology

Integrated care is essential when managing pediatric patients with complex congenital genitourinary anomalies. These children often require multispecialty therapies throughout their lives, necessitating the development of multidisciplinary teams that provide effective care.[13] A comprehensive example of multidisciplinary pediatric care is the Nationwide Children's Hospital Center for Colorectal and Pelvic Reconstruction. At this multidisciplinary clinic (MDC), pediatric patients

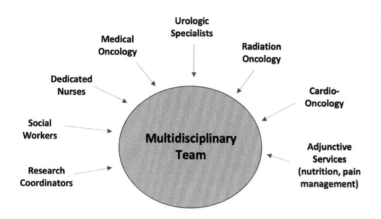

**Fig. 1.** Components of multidisciplinary teams in urology.

with anorectal malformations are seen in interdisciplinary clinics by specialists in pediatric urology, colorectal disease, gynecology, and gastroenterology and by psychologists, pelvic floor physical therapists, and social workers. For patients who require multiple surgical procedures, an attempt is made to coordinate cases among multiple surgical specialists to reduce hospital visits and anesthetic exposure. This integrated clinic model has been shown to decrease inpatient hospitalizations, clinic visits, rates of adverse anesthetic events, and health care costs and to improve the transition of care into adulthood.[14–16] Importantly, initiating these integrated clinics does not require a large upfront institutional investment and can financially benefit institutions relatively soon after implementation.[17]

### Female and Reconstructive Urology

Acquired, degenerative, and congenital neurourological disorders such as cerebrovascular injury, spinal cord injury, multiple sclerosis, Parkinson disease, spina bifida, and cerebral palsy often are associated with urinary, bowel, and sexual dysfunction. Coordinating these patients' care can optimize quality of life and health outcomes.[18] For example, spina bifida clinics are well described as improving patient outcomes by coordinating care from specialties such as orthopedics, neurosurgery, urology, psychiatry, nursing, social work, and physical/occupational therapists. Most of these patients require lifelong care for optimal life expectancy.[19]

Interstitial cystitis/bladder pain syndrome (IC/BPS) is one of the most challenging symptom complexes that urologists manage. The syndrome comprises a range of urinary symptoms, including pelvic pain, symptoms in nonpelvic organs, and psychological manifestations. Due to their heterogeneous symptoms, patients often

have seen multiple providers and have received numerous treatments that have failed to achieve adequate symptom control. To address this problem, Beaumont Health created a comprehensive Women's Urology and Pelvic Health Center composed of urologists who are experts in IC/BPS, gynecologists who manage female sexual dysfunction, colorectal surgeons who manage bowel dysfunction, pelvic floor physical therapists, and pain psychologists. Patients also can access acupuncture, medical massage, and nerve blocks provided by anesthesia pain providers. This integrative care model enables the clinic to successfully manage a complex condition by tailoring therapy to individual patients, which has resulted in better symptom management and patient satisfaction.[20] This is a good example of how integrative care works.

### Complex Genitourinary Oncology Care

Genitourinary malignancies, including cancers of prostate, kidney, bladder, testicle, and penis, are the most common cancers worldwide, and demand for genitourinary cancer care continues to increase amid global population aging.[21] Nowhere has the integrated care model in urology been better suited or studied than in urologic oncology. MDCs have become the new norm for oncologic care, and some experts even contend that this model should become the standard of care. We describe the implementation and structure of these MDCs and how they relate to patient care.

### MULTIDISCIPLINARY CLINIC MODELS IN UROLOGY

In general, MDCs in urologic oncology involve sequential same-day or concurrent visits to multiple providers at one location. This model aims to reduce patients' burden of care (ie, time, transportation difficulties, and costs), increase their understanding of their disease and treatment options, and mitigate challenges involved in specialist referrals to enhance patients' participation in shared decision making and evidence-based treatment. MDCs facilitate open communication about the risks and benefits of various treatment options and promote informed, collaborative decision making among patients and providers with the ultimate goal of individualizing treatment.[22]

Ideally, MDCs involve specialists in urologic oncology, radiation oncology, and medical oncology and offer adjunctive services from wound care and pain management specialists, nutritionists, pharmacists, psychologists, and social workers. Real-time input from radiologists and pathologists also provides invaluable information to guide patient care and management. Patients also are more likely to participate in research and clinical trials when treated in MDCs. Patients whose urologic malignancies are treated at high-volume MDC centers are reported to have better treatment outcomes compared with patients treated in noncentralized care facilities.[23]

## Tumor Boards

Weekly multidisciplinary team meetings or tumor boards are a vital component of MDCs in urologic oncology. Tumor boards usually comprise representatives from each oncology specialty (surgery, radiation oncology, and medical oncology), often with the addition of genitourinary-focused radiologists and pathologists. Cases are presented in a constructive and collaborative setting. Studies have linked the use of tumor boards with significant improvements in clinical and oncologic outcomes.[24]

Tumor boards can particularly benefit patients with advanced genitourinary malignancies and those requiring multimodal care.[24] In a prospective study of 296 patients with newly diagnosed urologic malignancies, treatment plans changed in 65% of cases after they were discussed at the weekly genitourinary tumor board.[25] Treatment changed most frequently in bladder cancer (44%), followed by kidney cancer (36%), testicular cancer (29%), and prostate cancer (22%). The ability of multidisciplinary tumor boards to alter management and tailor care is key for improving patient outcomes.

## Bladder Cancer

Bladder cancer is the fifth most common cancer and annually comprises approximately 450,000 new cases and 165,000 deaths globally.[26] One-third of these patients will present with advanced disease. Although MDCs can theoretically improve care for all stages and grades of bladder cancer, the management of muscle-invasive bladder cancer (MIBC) particularly stands to benefit. Patients with MIBC tend to be older (their average age is approximately 73 years) and to have comorbidities. Hence, shared decision making is critical, particularly because treatment involves the use of invasive and potentially morbid modalities. MDCs help foster effective communication among patients and providers regarding the risks and benefits of various treatment options.

Unfortunately, population-based studies indicate that only 50% of patients with MIBC receive curative treatment modalities such as radical cystectomy or trimodal bladder-sparing therapy.[27] Even more unsettling is the fact that only 21% of patients receive neoadjuvant chemotherapy before cystectomy, despite level 1 evidence of its benefit.[28,29] A lack of timely referrals to appropriate tertiary centers or specialty services contributes to these deficits. Collaboration within an MDC mitigates the challenges of cross-specialty referrals, which may increase the use of curative therapies for MIBC. Prior studies also indicate that centralizing patients' care in high-volume centers improves the utilization of radical cystectomy and decreases morbidity and mortality associated with surgery.[23]

Although we are still early in the development of MDCs in bladder cancer, some published data imply that this model can improve care. In one study of an MDC, imaging and pathology review of outside records and additional imaging ordered during multidisciplinary evaluation altered bladder cancer staging and treatment recommendations in 36% and 33% of patients, respectively.[30] In a study of 233 patients seen over 3 years at a tertiary medical center, the use of a bladder cancer MDC altered imaging interpretation in 26% of cases, changed pathologic interpretation in 29% of cases, changed recommendations for further workup in 42% of cases, altered clinical staging in 28% of cases, and led to treatment modifications in 58% of cases..[31] In a third study, the percentage of patients who received standard-of-care neoadjuvant chemotherapy increased from 7.7% at baseline to 47.6% after an MDC was implemented.[32]

## Prostate Cancer

Prostate cancer is the most common nonskin malignancy affecting men in the United States and the second leading cause of cancer mortality.[33] Despite this, the quality of prostate cancer treatment varies tremendously.[34] Most care continues to be delivered by local urologists working outside the setting of a specialized cancer center. In a recent retrospective study of more than 53,000 patients with prostate cancer who were recorded in a Surveillance Epidemiology and End Results (SEER)-Medicare database, there was considerable regional variation in practices such as pretreatment counseling by urologists and radiation oncologists, bone scans for patients with low-risk prostate cancer, combined androgen deprivation therapy and radiation therapy for patients with high-risk disease, and follow-up by radiation oncologists.[35] Variability in care may reflect variations in local physicians' knowledge of clinical guidelines and discrepant coordination among specialties such as urology and radiation oncology. These data, along with numerous prior studies documenting inconsistencies in prostate cancer care, argue for the creation of MDCs that manage both localized and advanced prostate cancer. We outline successful integrated care clinics for both these disease settings.

## Localized Prostate Cancer

Patients with low or intermediate-risk localized prostate cancer can potentially access the full gamut of options for management ranging from active surveillance, surgery, and radiotherapy to less common focal therapies such as high-intensity focused ultrasound or cryotherapy. Low and intermediate-risk disease is associated with high rates of survival regardless of treatment modality, but complications and decrements in quality of life vary widely. Given the number of treatment options with equivocal survival, it is key that patients fully understand each modality's risks and benefits so they can choose appropriate treatment. Treatment regret has been described in patients with prostate cancer, with up to 18% reporting that they regretted their treatment choice.[36]

Studies of MDCs in prostate cancer have demonstrated higher rates of patient satisfaction, more accurate classification of disease, and improved rates of survival and other desirable clinical outcomes as compared with studies of national cancer databases.[37–39] A successful clinic model has been described by Dr Leonard Gomella at the Sidney Kimmel Cancer Center at Jefferson Health.[39] At a weekly MDC, newly diagnosed patients with prostate cancer are seen by urologic surgical oncologists, radiation oncologists, medical oncologists, genitourinary pathologists, and dedicated oncology nurses and care coordinators. Appointments are scheduled for up to 60 minutes, allowing enough time for patients and families to speak with multiple specialists. The MDC model fosters real-time communication among a range of specialties during both the weekly clinic and the preclinic tumor board. More than 90% of patients have described their experience at this MDC as "good" or "very good." More than 15 years of experience at this MDC suggests that patients with prostate cancer benefit when they receive integrated care.

A multidisciplinary prostate cancer clinic helps patients become fully informed regarding all treatment options by making it easier for them to interact with multiple medical and surgical specialists. In one study, patients treated at a multidisciplinary prostate cancer clinic survived an average of 16.9 months longer compared with matched individuals from an SEER cohort.[40] In another study of 887 patients with newly diagnosed prostate cancer, 28.7% experienced a change in disease stage or risk category after they were seen at an MDC.[37] Using National Comprehensive Cancer Network guidelines as a benchmark, substantial proportions of patients were found to have previously received nonindicated bone scans (23.9%) and/or computed tomography/MRI studies (47.4%). In another study of 1031 patients with prostate cancer, management decisions differed significantly between those who participated in a multidisciplinary diagnostic assessment program and those who did not ($P<.0001$).[41]

## Advanced Prostate Cancer

Approximately 30% of patients with prostate cancer will develop metastatic disease.[42] Until recently, these patients had few treatment options, particularly after their disease became castration-resistant (mCRPC). In the not-so-distant era when mCRPC treatment was limited to cytotoxic chemotherapy, urologists often referred patients with mCRPC to medical oncology for further management. However, over the past 10 years, numerous treatment options have become available for patients with advanced prostate cancer. Urologists are now an integral part of the management of these patients and consequently have had to alter their practice structure to provide appropriate prostate cancer care within a rapidly changing treatment landscape.[43]

The recent expansion of treatment options for advanced prostate cancer heightens the need for multidisciplinary models in which urologists and oncologists collaborate to plan therapy, monitor treatment responses and adverse events, and adopt new treatments as needed.[44] Due to differences in training, urologists and medical oncologists tend to approach treatment decisions

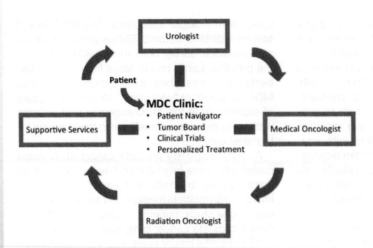

**Fig. 2.** MDC design in advanced prostate cancer.[43]

differently; also, patients with prostate cancer often are already established within a urology practice before their disease progresses and they require multidisciplinary treatment. These factors make it especially important to integrate care for advanced prostate cancer, either at a same-day, all-in-one clinic, or virtually through the use of tumor boards or messaging among providers. Key to this multidisciplinary approach is the use of shared managers who can evaluate new patient referrals and schedule visits with multiple providers concurrently.[43] **Fig. 2** demonstrates an example of MDC in advanced prostate cancer. Management should involve either weekly MDCs or tumor boards that perform multidisciplinary review. The MDC team should include genetic counselors, oncology-dedicated coordinators/nurses, research coordinators, nutritionists, social workers, and pain management specialists.

Multidisciplinary clinics tend to benefit patients with advanced prostate cancer, resulting in superior overall survival among patients with high-risk disease compared with national SEER data.[39,40] The advantage of MDCs in the treatment of advanced prostate cancer probably results from increased collaboration among subspecialists, the use of multidisciplinary tumor boards to confirm pathologic interpretation and management plans, and the use of evidence-based, state-of-the-art treatment modalities.

## Clinical Trials

Clinical oncology trials advance our understanding, treatment, and management of cancer but often suffer from low accrual rates. Surveys indicate that most patients with genitourinary malignancies are interested in participating in clinical research but are unaware of relevant trials and may not even know that participation is an option.[45] This is also true of many local urologists, who may be unfamiliar with different types of clinical trials and may lack the time to discuss trial enrollment.[46] Multidisciplinary clinics typically can offer longer appointment times and multispecialty counseling, which enables patients to receive more thorough counseling on clinical trials as well as coordinated recommendations from multiple providers.

## Palliation

Urologists often have long-term relationships with their patients, which uniquely positions them to facilitate hard discussions. Such trust and honest communication are especially important when it comes to discussions about palliative care for patients with metastatic genitourinary disease. Integrated urology and palliative care clinics have therefore been proposed. In a recent pilot study of such a clinic, patients reported improved patient and family satisfaction and were more likely to complete advanced care directives, maintain their quality of life, and die at home or at an inpatient hospice center.[47] A multidisciplinary approach at the end of life has obvious benefits for patients and has been shown to be feasible and well-received by providers.[48]

## Limitations of multidisciplinary centers

Throughout this article, we have described the benefits of integrated, multidisciplinary care. However, several potential disadvantages merit discussion. First, MDCs can be resource-intensive and time-consuming, especially during the early phase of development. Establishing an MDC requires a commitment by not only the institution or health care system, but also the providers and support staff. Coordinating schedules among busy providers is obviously challenging. Patients and families also may be overwhelmed or confused by the

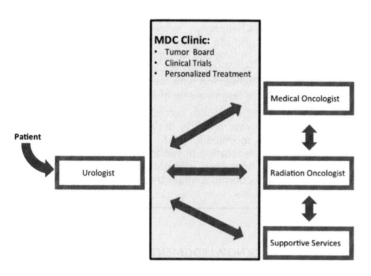

**Fig. 3.** Example of MDC virtual urologic oncology clinic.[43]

volume of information or counseling they receive at same-day MDCs. Limited space and lack of funding or staff to establish a comprehensive clinic have also been cited as barriers.[17] In the long-term, however, MDCs can be financially rewarding for both institutions and physicians.

### Implementation of integrated care in private practice

Most data on MDC models and outcomes come from studies of tertiary referral practices, such as large academic centers. However, many patients live far from these centers. In one study, patients were less likely to receive care at a multidisciplinary prostate cancer clinic if they lived more 100 miles from the center.[49] Although MDCs have been successfully implemented in community or private practice settings, they can be challenging to initiate in these environments due to the infrastructure and resources required. There also tends to be a higher margin of cost savings in community practices, and the very nature of MDCs can, at least initially, make them costly and time-consuming, especially in an already established busy private practice.

Experts recently described a strategy for integrating the management of complex genitourinary malignancies such as advanced prostate cancer.[50] They recommended that community practices designate leaders who will be responsible for the organization of the MDC, education of physician partners or other staff members, delegating responsibilities, and establishing in-person or virtual partnerships with other specialists. Developing integrated care models is especially important in regions that are underserved by subspecialists, such as genitourinary oncologists and urologic oncologists. In these areas, integrated

urologic care can improve access to treatment in general, as well as access to novel, evidence-based novel treatment modalities.[50]

### Future of integrated care

**Telemedicine** Until recently, technologies for remote communication such as telehealth visits and teleconsultation had not been widely implemented. Early studies of telehealth in urology have shown increased patient satisfaction and access to care and decreased health care costs.[51] However, physicians have been reluctant to adopt telemedicine due to the inherent challenges of implementing new technologies and the variable reimbursement environment.[52]

The Coronavirus Disease 2019 (COVID-19) pandemic has necessitated widespread and substantial changes in health care delivery, including the routine use of video visits, teleconsultations, and other forms of electronic communication. Physicians have had to rapidly adapt their practices, and there are no long-term data yet on how this transition has affected patient outcomes. However, in pre-pandemic studies of general urology practices, virtual visits were shown to be successful for managing urinary tract infections, uncomplicated urinary stones, incontinence, pelvic organ prolapse, and even uncomplicated, localized prostate cancer.[53]

So far, there have been only a few descriptions of virtual MDCs and tumor boards for genitourinary malignancies. However, they are an attractive option that could potentially surmount the barriers to implementing single-location MDCs, such as patient travel time, transportation costs, access to transport, and physician time and space limitations.[43] **Fig. 3** represents how a virtual genitourinary urologic oncology MDC can be organized. In a virtual cancer care model, patients might see a general provider nearby who helps coordinate oncologic care by communicating with other providers or with a multidisciplinary tumor board; however, successful implementation would require close communication among providers and staff. Virtual multidisciplinary tumor boards and teleconsultation are already occurring to facilitate social distancing during the COVID-19 pandemic. In all likelihood, the increased uptake of telemedicine will persist even after the pandemic ends.

## SUMMARY

Integrated care in urology is constantly evolving, but thus far has proven itself in terms of its benefits to patients and its ability to maintain reimbursements in the era of alternative payment models. Integrated care benefits all patients in urology, from pediatrics through transitional care and into adulthood. Multidisciplinary clinics have become the standard of care for managing patients with genitourinary malignancies. Implementing MDCs at both community and tertiary referral centers can be resource-intensive and time-consuming, but doing so can ultimately improve coordination of care and access to treatments that are likely to ultimately reduce long-term health care costs.

## CLINICS CARE POINTS

- The goal of integrated health care is to improve patient outcomes and experiences while reducing costs associated with a specific health care delivery.
- Integrated urologic care can particularly benefit patients who have complex pediatric genitourinary conditions, neuro-urologic disorders, interstitial cystitis or bladder pain syndrome, and complex urologic tumors.
- MDCs in urologic oncology typically offer sequential same-day or concurrent visits with multiple providers at one location. Ideally, these should include specialists in urologic oncology, radiation oncology, and medical oncology, as well as wound care and pain management specialists, nutritionists, pharmacists, psychologists, and social workers.
- Tumor boards are a vital part of MDCs in urologic oncology. Input from multiple specialists during case reviews frequently alters treatment plans and can improve clinical outcomes.

- Challenges when implementing MDCs include a considerable upfront investment of time and resources, the need to coordinate providers' schedules, and the risk of overwhelming patients and families by providing a large volume of information at once.
- To establish successful urology MDCs in private practice, designate leaders to take responsibility for organizing the MDC, educating physician partners and other staff members, delegating responsibilities, and coordinating partnerships with other specialists.

## ACKNOWLEDGMENTS

The authors thank Dr Amy Karon for editorial assistance.

## DISCLOSURE

Dr M. Cookson has advisory roles with Astellas, Bayer, Janssen, and Merck. Dr N. Shore has research/consulting roles with AbbVie, Amgen, AstraZeneca, Astellas, Bayer, BMS, Clovis Oncology, Dendreon, Exact Imaging, Exact Sciences, Fergene, Ferring, Janssen, MDxHealth, Merck, Myovant, Novartis, Nymox, Pantarhei, Pfizer, Sanofi-Genzyme, and Tolmar.

## REFERENCES

1. Lee TH, Bothe A, Steele GD. How Geisinger structures its physicians' compensation to support improvements in quality, efficiency, and volume. Health Aff (Millwood) 2012;31:2068–73.
2. Enthoven AC. Integrated delivery systems: the cure for fragmentation. Am J Manag Care 2009;15: S284–90.
3. Herrel LA, Kaufman SA, Yan P, et al. Health care integration and quality among men with prostate cancer. J Urol 2017;197:55–60.
4. Mittinty MM, Marshall A, Harvey G. What integrated care means from an older person's perspective? A scoping review protocol. BMJ Open 2018;8: e019256.
5. Kocot SL, White R, Tu T, et al. The impact of accountable care: origins and future of accountable care organizations. Available at: https://www.brookings.edu/research/the-impact-of-accountable-care-origins-and-future-of-accountable-care-organizations/. Accessed October 29, 2020.
6. Institute for Healthcare Improvement. The IHI triple aim. Available at: http://www.ihi.org/engage/initiatives/TripleAim/Pages/default.aspx. Accessed October 29, 2020.

7. Hawken SR, Herrel LA, Ellimoottil C, et al. Urologist participation in Medicare shared savings program accountable care organizations (ACOs). Urology 2016;90:76–80.

8. Soukup T, Lamb BW, Arora S, et al. Successful strategies in implementing a multidisciplinary team working in the care of patients with cancer: an overview and synthesis of the available literature. J Multidiscip Healthc 2018;11:49–61.

9. Horvath LE, Yordan E, Malhotra D, et al. Multidisciplinary care in the oncology setting: historical perspective and data from lung and gynecology multidisciplinary clinics. J Oncol Pract 2010;6:e21–6.

10. Newman EA, Guest AB, Helvie MA, et al. Changes in surgical management resulting from case review at a breast cancer multidisciplinary tumor board. Cancer 2006;107:2346–51.

11. Conron M, Phuah S, Steinfort D, et al. Analysis of multidisciplinary lung cancer practice. Intern Med J 2007;37:18–25.

12. Singh J, Fairbairn KJ, Williams C, et al. Expert radiological review of skeletal surveys identifies additional abnormalities in 23% of cases: further evidence for the value of myeloma multidisciplinary teams in the accurate staging and treatment of myeloma patients. Br J Haematol 2007;137:172–3.

13. Woodhouse CR, Neild GH, Yu RN, et al. Adult care of children from pediatric urology. J Urol 2012;187:1164–71.

14. Vilanova-Sanchez A, Halleran DR, Reck-Burneo CA, et al. A descriptive model for a multidisciplinary unit for colorectal and pelvic malformations. J Pediatr Surg 2019;54:479–85.

15. Lambert SM. Transitional care in pediatric urology. Semin Pediatr Surg 2015;24:73–8.

16. Vilanova-Sánchez A, Reck CA, Wood RJ, et al. Impact on patient care of a multidisciplinary center specializing in colorectal and pelvic reconstruction. Front Surg 2018;5:68.

17. Style CC, Hsu DM, Verla MA, et al. Development of a multidisciplinary colorectal and pelvic health program: program implementation and clinical impact. J Pediatr Surg 2020;55(11):2397–402.

18. Agrawal S, Agrawal RR, Wood HM. Establishing a multidisciplinary approach to the management of neurologic disease affecting the urinary tract. Urol Clin North Am 2017;44:377–89.

19. Groen J, Pannek D, Castro Diaz D, et al. Summary of European Association of Urology (EAU) guidelines on neuro-urology. Eur Urol 2016;69:324–33.

20. Gupta P, Gaines N, Sirls LT, et al. A multidisciplinary approach to the evaluation and management of interstitial cystitis/bladder pain syndrome: an ideal model of care. Transl Androl Urol 2015;4:611–9.

21. Dy DW, Gore JL, Forouzanfar MH, et al. Global burden of urologic cancers, 1990-2013. Eur Urol 2017;71:437–46.

22. Harshman L, Tripathi A, Kaag M, et al. Contemporary patterns of multidisciplinary care in patients with muscle-invasive bladder cancer. Clin Genitour Cancer 2018;16:213–8.

23. Williams SB, Ray-Zack MD, Hudgins HK, et al. Impact of centralizing care for genitourinary malignancies to high-volume providers: a systematic review. Eur Urol Oncol 2019;2(3):265–73.

24. Rao K, Manya K, Azad A, et al. Uro-oncology multidisciplinary meetings at an Australian tertiary referral centre–impact on clinical decision-making and implications for patient inclusion. BJU Int 2014;114(Suppl 1):50–4.

25. Kurpad R, Kim W, Rathmell WK, et al. A multidisciplinary approach to the management of urologic malignancies: does it influence diagnostic and treatment decisions? Urol Oncol 2011;29(4):378–82.

26. McGuire S. World Cancer Report 2014. Geneva, Switzerland. World Health Organization. International Agency for Research on Cancer. WHO Press, 2015. Adv Nutr 2016;7:418–9.

27. Gray PJ, Fedewa SA, WU Shipley, et al. Use of potentially curative therapies for muscle-invasive bladder cancer in the United States: results from the National Cancer Database. Eur Urol 2013;63:823–9.

28. Zaid HB, Patel SG, Stimson CJ, et al. Trends in the utilization of neoadjuvant chemotherapy in muscle-invasive bladder cancer: results from the National Cancer Database. Urology 2014;83:75–80.

29. Reardon ZD, Patel SG, Zaid HB, et al. Trends in the use of perioperative chemotherapy for localized and locally advanced muscle-invasive bladder cancer: a sign of changing tides. Eur Urol 2015;67:165–70.

30. Kulkarni GS, Hermanns T, Wei Y, et al. Propensity score analysis of radical cystectomy versus bladder-sparing trimodal therapy in the setting of a multidisciplinary bladder cancer clinic. J Clin Oncol 2017;35:2299–305.

31. Diamantopoulos LN, Winters BR, Grivas P, et al. Bladder cancer multidisciplinary clinic (BCMC) model influences disease assessment and impacts treatment recommendations. Bladder Cancer 2019;5:289–98.

32. Nayan M, Bhindi B, Yu JL, et al. The initiation of a multidisciplinary bladder cancer clinic and the uptake of neoadjuvant chemotherapy: A time-series analysis. Can Urol Assoc J 2016;10:25–30.

33. Jemal A, Siegel R, Xu J, et al. Cancer statistics, 2010. CA Cancer J Clin 2010;60:277–300.

34. Schroeck FR, Kaufman SR, Jacobs BL, et al. Regional variation in quality of prostate cancer care. J Urol 2014;191:957–62.

35. Zapka J, Taplin SH, Ganz P, et al. Multilevel factors affecting quality: examples from the cancer care continuum. J Natl Cancer Inst Monogr 2012;2012: 11–9.

36. Hu JC, Kwan L, Krupski TL, et al. Determinants of treatment regret in low-income, uninsured men with prostate cancer. Urology 2008;72:1274–9.

37. Sundi D, Cohen JE, Cole AP, et al. Establishment of a new prostate cancer multidisciplinary clinic: Format and initial experience. Prostate 2015;75: 191–9.

38. Hong NJ, Wright FC, Gagliardi AR, et al. Examining the potential relationship between multidisciplinary cancer care and patient survival: an international literature review. J Surg Oncol 2010;102:125–34.

39. Gomella LG, Lin J, Hoffman-Censits J, et al. Enhancing prostate cancer care through the multidisciplinary clinic approach: a 15-year experience. J Oncol Pract 2010;6:e5–10.

40. Reichard CA, Hoffman KE, Tang C, et al. Radical prostatectomy or radiotherapy for high- and very high-risk prostate cancer: a multidisciplinary prostate cancer clinic experience of patients eligible for either treatment. BJU Int 2019;124:811–9.

41. Guy D, Ghanem G, Loblaw A, et al. Diagnosis, referral, and primary treatment decisions in newly diagnosed prostate cancer patients in a multidisciplinary diagnostic assessment program. Can Urol Assoc J 2016;10:120–5.

42. Pound CR, Partin AW, Eisenberger MA, et al. Natural history of progression after PSA elevation following radical prostatectomy. JAMA 1999;281:1591–7.

43. Stratton KL, Moeller AM, Cookson MS. Implementation of the AUA castration resistant prostate cancer guidelines into practice: establishing a multidisciplinary clinic. Urol Pract 2016;3:203–9.

44. Sartor AO, Fitzpatrick JM. Urologists and oncologists: adapting to a new treatment paradigm in castration-resistant prostate cancer (CRPC). BJU Int 2012;110:328–35.

45. Madsen LT, Kuban DA, Choi S, et al. Impact of a clinical trial initiative on clinical trial enrollment in a multidisciplinary prostate cancer clinic. J Natl Compr Canc Netw 2014;12:993–8.

46. Jacobs SR, Weiner BJ, Minasian LM, et al. Achieving high cancer control trial enrollment in the community setting: an analysis of the Community Clinical Oncology Program. Contemp Clin Trials 2013;34:320–5.

47. Huen K, Huang C, Liu H, et al. Outcomes of an integrated urology-palliative care clinic for patients with advanced urological cancers: maintenance of quality of life and satisfaction and high rate of hospice utilization through end of life. Am J Hosp Palliat Care 2019;36:801–6.

48. Bergman J, Ballon-Landa E, Lorenz KA, et al. Community-partnered collaboration to build an integrated palliative care clinic: the view from urology. Am J Hosp Palliat Care 2016;33:164–70.

49. Stewart SB, Bañez LL, Robertson CN, et al. Utilization trends at a multidisciplinary prostate cancer clinic: initial 5-year experience from the Duke Prostate Center. J Urol 2012;187:103–8.

50. Shore N. Management of advanced prostate cancer - role of the urologist. Curr Urol Rep 2014;15:419.

51. Rumaihi KA, Boorjian SA, Jewett M. Evolving changes in the delivery of health services: a place for urological homecare? Eur Urol 2019;75:543–5.

52. Gadzinski AJ, Ellimoottil C. Telehealth in urology after the COVID-19 pandemic. Nat Rev Urol 2020;17: 363–4.

53. Novara G, Checcucci E, Crestani A, et al. Telehealth in urology: a systematic review of the literature. How much can telemedicine be useful during and after the COVID-19 pandemic? Eur Urol 2020;78(6): 786–811.

# Private Equity and Urology
## An Emerging Model for Independent Practice

Gary M. Kirsh, MD[a],*, Deepak A. Kapoor, MD[b]

## KEYWORDS

- Urology • Private equity • Consolidation • Health care

## KEY POINTS

- Urology practices motivated to remain independent are under mounting competitive and operational pressures, and large hospital systems continue to acquire physicians.
- Private equity can help independent urology practices grow and consolidate so that they can better implement best practices, unleash new revenue opportunities, and more effectively compete in the marketplace.
- Independent urology practices seeking private equity investment should carefully consider the benefits of private equity and understand the private equity transaction structure.

## EXECUTIVE SUMMARY

Driven by regulatory developments, market forces, and sweeping structural changes, consolidation has been a dominant trend in health care over more than a decade. From hospital systems to insurance providers to physician practices ranging from dermatology to ophthalmology to dentistry, all corners of health care are consolidating, with larger superregional and national players quickly becoming the norm, and urology is no exception.

Independent urology practices are under increasing competitive pressure, as hospitals seek to acquire more physicians to strengthen their own positions in the face of a changing marketplace and meet the needs of patients. In response, independent urology clinicians have formed regional groups that allow for greater economies of scale, better access to ancillary services, and more efficiency in navigating an increasingly complex reimbursement and regulatory landscape.

Now independent urology is at a critical inflection point as it transitions from a regional model to a national model. A key factor in this stage of development is the use of private equity. By providing access to capital, as well as operational resources and business management expertise, private equity can act as a powerful lever. Urology practices that partner with private equity can better scale to compete with large hospital systems, while unlocking new growth opportunities, maintaining clinical excellence, and, critically, allowing physicians to retain ownership, the sine qua non of independence, with the added opportunity for equity appreciation.

Although some practice owners may still choose neither the hospital nor private equity route and would rather go it alone, this path is an increasingly difficult one to follow and is by no means a certain recipe for success. Now, more than ever, health care is a dynamic market, where there is no such thing as the status quo. With technology-enabled disruptors, the volatility of the payer market, and new care delivery models, there are few areas of certainty. Doing nothing to evolve is an active decision that also carries risk.

[a] The Urology Group Cincinnati, Solaris Health Holdings, 2000 Joseph E. Sanker Boulevard, Cincinnati, OH 45212, USA; [b] Integrated Medical Professionals, Solaris Health Holdings, LLC, The Icahn School of Medicine at Mount Sinai, 340 Broadhollow Road, Farmingdale, NY 11735, USA
* Corresponding author.
*E-mail address:* gkirsh@urologygroup.com

Urol Clin N Am 48 (2021) 233–244
https://doi.org/10.1016/j.ucl.2020.12.004

In this article, the authors take a close look at the forces driving consolidation across the health care industry, and urology specifically, as well as the challenges that independent urology practices face. They also examine how private equity firms operate and what their position is in the urology marketplace. In addition, the authors explore the potential benefits of private equity investment, what firms look for in investment partners, how to prepare your organization for private equity investment, and the structure of a typical private equity-backed managed services organization (MSO).

## HEALTH CARE INDUSTRY CONSOLIDATION AND INDEPENDENT PHYSICIAN PRACTICES

Over the past decade, the health care industry has undergone a wave of consolidation affecting nearly every type of organization and specialty, regardless of size. A recent study published in Bloomberg Law[1] (**Fig. 1**) found that health care consolidation across nearly all corners of the industry remained robust in 2019, with a total of 1588 deals closed or announced. Physician practice acquisition ranked second only to long-term care in the number of transactions conducted.

As a result, the health care landscape has been radically transformed, and the process is still underway.

One major factor accelerating consolidation over the past decade is the 2010 passage of the Affordable Care Act (ACA). The ACA had several far-reaching impacts, among them the increase of accountable care organizations (ACOs) under the Medicare program. The logic behind ACOs was that doctors, hospitals, and other health care providers that formed networks could better coordinate patient care and deliver that care more efficiently.

Although ACOs have not taken off as many proponents of the ACA legislation contemplated, and the number of Medicare ACOs has remained relatively flat,[2] they have nevertheless had a profound impact on health systems and the continued survival of independent medical practices. The drive toward ACOs served as a spark for further changes, including hospital systems buying physician practices to capture the legions of doctors needed to effectively serve newly covered lives.

According to Avalere Health and the Physicians Advisory Institute, between 2016 and 2018, hospitals acquired 8000 medical practices, while 14,000 physicians left private practice to work in hospitals.[3]

The hospital threat to independent physician practices comprises several interconnected factors that make it more challenging than ever for doctors to maintain autonomy. These factors include increasingly complex government

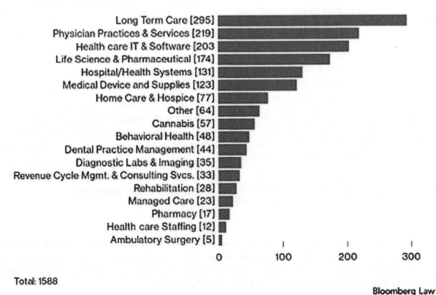

**Fig. 1.** Health care consolidation across practice areas. IT, information technology; Mgmt., management; Svcs., services. (*From* Bloomberg Law. Published Jan. 27, 2020. Copyright 2020 by The Bureau of National Affairs, Inc. (800-372-1033) <http://www.bloombergindustry.com>; with permission.)

regulations and reimbursement rules, the prospect of financial buyouts from hospital systems, the potential lack of referrals from primary care doctors within hospitals' systems, and the threat that hospital networks may hire "their own" physicians if independent practitioners fail to fall in line and agree to be acquired.

However, hospital system growth is not the only threat to independence. Large insurance companies are also venturing into the provider side of health care. UnitedHealth Group's Optum division recently acquired Surgical Care Affiliates for $2.3 billion,[4] establishing a base for Optimate's primary and specialty care division, which focuses on acquiring or partnering with private medical practices.

## THE EVOLUTION OF INDEPENDENT UROLOGY PRACTICES

Like practitioners across several other specialty areas, urologists wishing to maintain their independence in the post-ACA environment face increasing headwinds, which take many forms: administrative costs, reimbursement complexity, a lack of leverage in negotiations with large payers, competition in recruitment, and the need for increasingly sophisticated business services, including management, legal, accounting, information technology, and human resources.

The impact of these challenges has been dramatic, with 46% of urologists now employed by hospitals and institutions, whereas the percentage of urologists in private practice decreased by approximately 10% from 2015 to 2019, from 63% to 53%, according to the latest 2019 AUA census data.[5]

Today, 5118[5] urologists are either solo practitioners or part of independent single-specialty urology groups, but the market remains highly fragmented. According to Brighter Health Network, the 5 largest specialty urology groups in the country employ approximately 468 providers, including nurse practitioners, physicians' assistants, urogynecologists, and oncologists, representing 9% of the total. Moreover, only 7 practices nationally have more than 50 total providers (**Table 1**).[6]

This flight of urologists from private practices to hospital networks is taking place against the backdrop of a long-term evolution in the structure of independent urology practices that predates the ACA, is driven by several complex forces, and can be thought about in following 3 broad stages (**Fig. 2**).

### The Historic Practice Era

Throughout the twentieth century and well into the early to mid-1990s, urology, like many other

**Table 1**
**Largest specialty urology groups in United States**

| Size Rank | Practice Name | Number of Urologists |
|---|---|---|
| 1 | Solaris Health Holdings | 182 |
| 2 | United Urology Group | 161 |
| 3 | 21st Century Oncology | 121 |
| 4 | New Jersey Urology | 119 |
| 5 | Southern California Permanente Medical Group | 99 |
| 6 | Permanente Medical Group Inc | 89 |
| 7 | Advanced Urology Institute | 68 |
| 8 | Cleveland Clinic Foundation | 64 |
| 9 | University Of Pittsburgh Physicians | 53 |
| 10 | Uropartners | 52 |
| 11 | Georgia Urology | 49 |
| 12 | Mayo Clinic | 49 |
| 13 | North Shore-LIJ Medical | 49 |
| 14 | US Urology | 47 |
| 15 | Urology Clinics Of North Texas | 43 |
| 16 | Regents Of The University Of Michigan | 41 |
| 17 | Michigan Institute Of Urology | 40 |
| 18 | Michigan Healthcare Professionals | 37 |
| 19 | Minnesota Urology | 36 |
| 20 | Virginia Urology Center | 33 |

*Data from* Medicare Data on Physician Practice and Specialty (MD-PPAS), individual group website provider count;2017.

specialty areas, was characterized by hundreds of small practices. These practices typically consisted of between 1 and 5 physicians focused on serving a limited, local market. During this period, which the authors call the "historic practice era," physician revenue was almost exclusively driven by the direct provision of evaluative or surgical care to patients.

### Emergence and Proliferation of Regional Leaders

Beginning in the early 1990s, larger regional urology practices began to emerge. The market

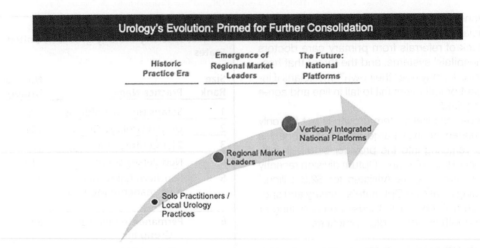

**Fig. 2.** Waves of consolidation in urology.

dynamics behind this shift are multifaceted. One important initial driver was the need for better negotiating power with payers as compensation for professional services decreased, and urologists saw that they were earning progressively lower revenues from their personal interactions with patients. To compensate, many independent practices sought new revenue streams through the addition of services unrelated to the direct provision of care. Beginning with capabilities such as ambulatory service centers (ASCs) and then progressing to imaging, laboratory, clinical research, radiation, and pharmacy, the last 3 decades have seen a steady increase in these and other ancillary services.

These more powerful regional practices came together primarily through mergers. A natural evolution of the formation of these regional leaders was the establishment of the nonprofit urology trade association Large Urology Group Practice Association (LUGPA), which has fostered increased interaction and networking among independent urology groups and further driven growth. As a result, the percentage of private practice urologists working in large groups consisting of 10 providers or more grew from 15% in 2015 to 32% in 2019.[5]

## The Future: National Urology Platforms

As external pressures on independent practices have increased, this second stage has "primed the pump" for regional leaders to consider national consolidation and partnership to achieve greater scale.

The vision behind larger-scale *national* platforms is a linking of large regional groups that avoids the need to "reinvent the wheel" in each geography and provides resources that smaller regional practices cannot access on their own. Factors driving urologists to consider the formation of national platforms include the following factors.

### Regulatory considerations

For urologists, it has become increasingly difficult to manage the regulatory burden of administering a practice in a silo. The enactment of the Medicare Access and CHIP Reauthorization Act of 2015 and its MIPS program, the specter of emerging "alternative payment models" (including Centers for Medicare & Medicaid Services' recently announced radiation oncology alternative payment model), and electronic records rules are just 3 examples of complex regulations that require time and resources to manage. The cumulative effect can be profound and takes physician attention away from building practices and serving patients.

### Operational efficiency

National networks can accelerate the operational and quality-of-care benefits gained through sharing of best practices and centralizing costly back office and administrative functions, such as human resources, legal, accounting, revenue cycle management, and information technology. According to Medscape, urologists spend an average of 15.1 hours per week just on paperwork and administrative tasks.[7]

### Clinical burdens and subspecialization

As the practice of medicine becomes more complicated and the volume of clinical information continues to expand, it has become harder for urologists to be good at everything. With national scale, urologists are better able to define clinical pathways and best practices in subspecialty areas and disseminate that information out to the national network.

### Revenue opportunities

A national practice entity can provide the assistance needed for local practices to implement revenue enhancing ancillary revenue streams if they have not had the wherewithal to do so previously. Moreover, national scale may provide even sophisticated practices with an opportunity to unlock new revenue opportunities not previously accessible, such as leveraging proprietary practice data and other clinical resources, development of win-win value-based reimbursement models, as well as other sources not yet envisioned.

As the US health care system continues to rapidly evolve and the pressure on non-hospital-affiliated urology practices increases, national consolidation at scale may be the only way for urologists to compete while retaining their independence. However, these increased demands necessitate capital, expertise, and resources beyond the means of even large regional players, creating a natural entry point for private equity.

## ENTER PRIVATE EQUITY

With nearly $600 billion raised in 2019,[8] across a broad range of industries and strategies, private equity firms play a critical role in the global economy and in investors' portfolios. At the beginning of 2020, Preqin estimated[9] that private equity investors were sitting on a record amount, $1.45 trillion, in "dry powder," or cash available to invest.

To understand why private equity has grown to become such a major force in the global economy, it is important to understand how it works.

Private equity is often categorized as an "alternative investment." That is to say that it is an alternative to the stock and bond portfolios traditionally used by investors. Private equity seeks to earn returns that are better than what can be achieved in public equity markets through an expanded opportunity set of investments not typically available through public markets, legitimate access to nonpublic information before making an investment, a strong alignment of interests, and a greater degree of control and influence over investments. Over the past 30 years, US private equity has delivered greater average net returns compared with an alternative private-market performance benchmark using the S&P 500 as the proxy.[10]

Generally speaking, private equity firms raise pools of capital known as funds, from a variety of investors, commonly high-net-worth individuals or families, corporate and public pensions, endowments, and foundations. These funds are structured as limited partnerships comprising the firm, known as the General Partner (GP), and the investors, known as Limited Partners (LPs).

It is the GP's job to identify quality companies with growth potential, invest in them, and grow their value. Achieving these goals can involve much more than just providing capital. GPs serve as advisors to portfolio company management, helping to streamline operations, develop productive leadership teams, and identify new avenues for growth.

Typically, after 3 to 7 years of ownership, the GP will seek to "exit" the company by taking the business public or selling it to another private equity firm or corporation. This exit distributes profits from the sale ("returns") to the investors in the private equity fund, the fund manager, any other investors in the company, and, in the case of physician practices, the physician shareholders.

Although all private equity firms follow this general approach, there are many variations based on size of investment, timing of investment, and other factors. For example, "venture capital" denotes firms making a greater number of less certain and relatively smaller investments in early-stage companies. "Growth equity" often designates a firm that takes minority stakes in mid-stage companies, and "buyout" most often refers to firms that purchase a majority stake of the businesses they invest in, through a combination of equity and debt financing.

Although the largest private equity firms can have funds of more than $10 billion, most of the industry is composed of "middle market" firms managing funds with capital commitments between $100 million and $5 billion and focusing on transactions valued between $25 million and $1 billion.[11] According to PitchBook, in quarter 1 2020, 27 middle-market funds raised $24.81 billion of capital.[12] Middle market buyout firms are those most likely to be interested in urology practice investments.

## PRIVATE EQUITY IN HEALTH CARE

In recent years, private equity has emerged as a major engine of growth across the health care landscape. According to Bain & Company's *Global Healthcare Private Equity and Corporate M&A Report 2020*,[13] more than $79 billion was invested by private equity in the sector globally in 2019, the highest on record and a 5-fold increase over the previous 10 years. North American health care deal value in 2019 reached an all-time high of $46.7 billion, whereas health care deal volume increased from 149 in 2018 to 159 in 2019.[13]

Private equity's interest in health care is due in part to the sector's resiliency through macroeconomic cycles. The often inefficient, siloed, and fragmented nature of health delivery is also a natural match for private equity's ability to enhance value by helping to streamline inefficiencies, develop productive leadership teams, improve operating models, and find new avenues for growth.

Another factor in private equity's enduring interest in the health care sector is that it continues to exhibit viable paths to seek full or partial liquidity, so investment proceeds can be distributed to LPs. The ability to have a partial or full exit event is increasing. More than 100 health care private equity platforms are sold by 1 financial sponsor or private equity firm to another each year. Sixty percent of these exits are sales to larger private equity firms, whereas 5% to 10% are initial public offerings (**Fig. 3**).[13]

Furthermore, as Ernst & Young's *May 2020 Health Global Capital Confidence Barometer*[14] underscores, the COVID-19 pandemic has amplified the need for health care industry improvements and the investment they require, with health care management teams' expectations for mergers and acquisitions (M&A) in 2020 increasing to a 10-year high (**Fig. 4**).[15] Hospitals and health care providers, among the sectors most impacted by the pandemic, will need to be agile to reshape and reinvent themselves for the future, opening the door to strategic M&A.

The provider and related services segment has accounted for the greatest number of health care

private equity deals to date, with 96 in 2019, up from 84 in 2018 (**Fig. 5**).[13]

According to a February 2020 *The Journal of the American Medical Association* (*JAMA*) Study[16] of private equity medical group acquisitions between 2013 and 2016, the groups with the highest rates of private equity backing include anesthesiology (19.4%), multispecialty (19.4%), emergency medicine (12.1%), family practice (11.0%), and dermatology (9.9%). From 2015 to 2016, there was also an increase in the number of acquired cardiology, ophthalmology, radiology, and obstetrics/gynecology practices.

With the shift to value-based care, private equity firms are increasingly interested in specialties that both have independent private practices and present opportunities to consolidate regional markets and build industry leaders with defensible market positions (**Fig. 6**). The *JAMA* report cited above bears this out, showing the number of private equity deals with physician practices across specialties more than doubled between 2013 and 2016.[16]

## PRIVATE EQUITY INTEREST IN UROLOGY

Given the context provided above, it should come as no surprise that private equity has turned its attention to urology in the United States, where the growth prospects are strong, and there are more than 13,000 practicing physicians as of 2019, 53% of whom are in private practice.[5]

Driven in large part by increases in longevity, the demand for urologic care has never been higher, as conditions such as prostate cancer, urinary incontinence, and benign prostatic hyperplasia

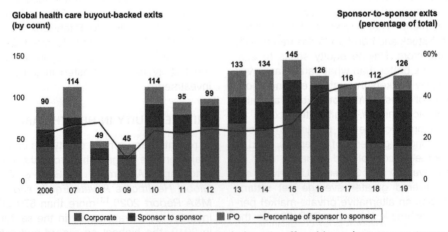

**Fig. 3.** Global private equity health care exits. Notes: Excludes spin-offs, add-ons, loan-to-own transactions and acquisitions of bankrupt assets; based on announcement date; includes announced deals that are completed or pending, with data subject to change; deal values does not account for deals with undisclosed values. Sources: Dealogic; AVCJ; Bain analysis. (*Used with permission* from Bain & Company.)

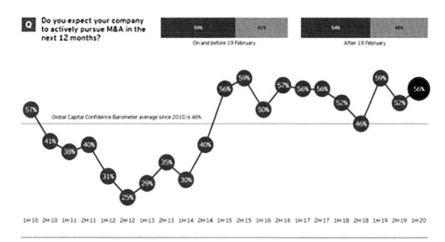

**Fig. 4.** Health care M&A expectations: 2020. (*From* EYGM Limited. © 2020 EYGM Limited. All Rights Reserved. <https://assets.ey.com/content/dam/ey-sites/ey-com/en_gl/topics/ey-capital-confidence-barometer/pdfs/22/ey-22nd-global-capital-confidence-barometer-march-2020.pdf>; with permission.)

increase among the growing over-60 population. According to a recent Provident study,[17] this demand is currently on pace to outstrip the supply of urologists.

More than half of the practicing urologists in the United States, or 6175 urologists, are over the age of 55, with approximately just 300 graduating from residency programs each year. This gap between physician supply and patient demand ensures a steady stream of business for urologists and makes urology especially attractive for private equity.

Equally attractive for private equity investors are 2 important factors. First is the opportunity that urology offers to consolidate a fragmented market. Second, urology offers the ability to add on ancillary services referenced above, along the continuum of patient care, creating diversified revenue streams.

Several private equity groups have partnered with leading platforms in the urology sector and are likely to continue to consolidate fragmented regional markets through add-on acquisitions. Examples include Audax Group's 2016 investment in Chesapeake Urology; J.W. Childs Associates formation of Urology Management Associates with New Jersey Urology in 2018; NMS Capital's funding of US Urology Partners in 2019; and Lee Equity

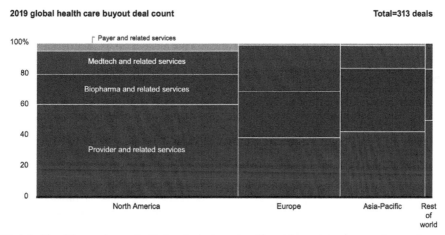

**Fig. 5.** 2019 global health care buyouts. Notes: Excludes spin-offs, add-ons, loan-to-own transactions and acquisitions of bankrupt assets; based on announcement date; includes announced deals that are completed or pending, with data subject to change; deal values does not account for deals with undisclosed values; geography based on the location of targets. Sources: Dealogic; AVCJ; Bain analysis. (*Used with permission* from Bain & Company.)

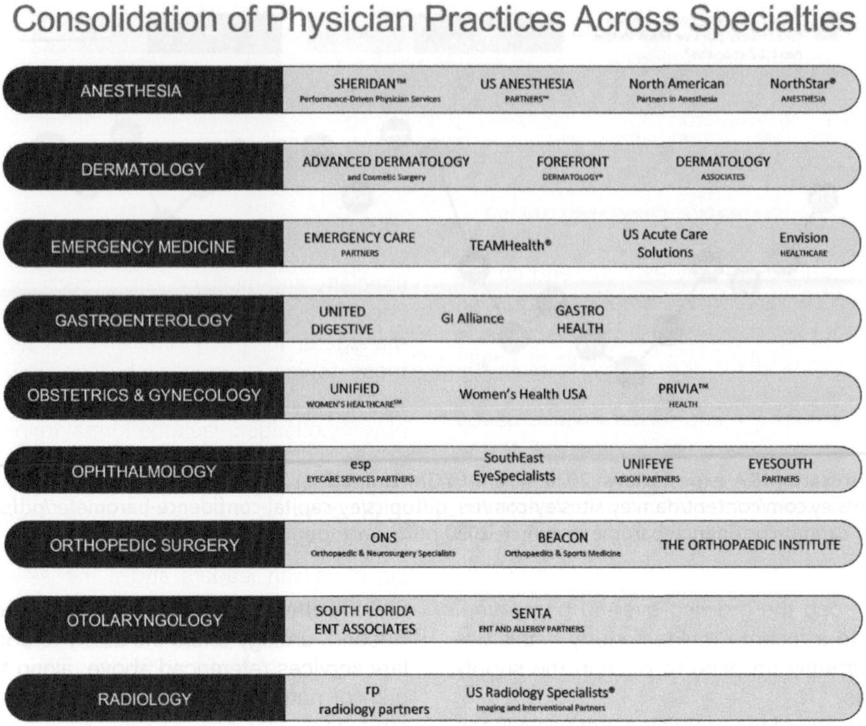

## Consolidation of Physician Practices Across Specialties

| ANESTHESIA | SHERIDAN™ Performance-Driven Physician Services | US ANESTHESIA PARTNERS™ | North American Partners in Anesthesia | NorthStar® ANESTHESIA |
|---|---|---|---|---|
| DERMATOLOGY | ADVANCED DERMATOLOGY and Cosmetic Surgery | FOREFRONT DERMATOLOGY® | DERMATOLOGY ASSOCIATES | |
| EMERGENCY MEDICINE | EMERGENCY CARE PARTNERS | TEAMHealth® | US Acute Care Solutions | Envision HEALTHCARE |
| GASTROENTEROLOGY | UNITED DIGESTIVE | GI Alliance | GASTRO HEALTH | |
| OBSTETRICS & GYNECOLOGY | UNIFIED WOMEN'S HEALTHCARE℠ | Women's Health USA | PRIVIA™ HEALTH | |
| OPHTHALMOLOGY | esp EYECARE SERVICES PARTNERS | SouthEast EyeSpecialists | UNIFEYE VISION PARTNERS | EYESOUTH PARTNERS |
| ORTHOPEDIC SURGERY | ONS Orthopaedic & Neurosurgery Specialists | BEACON Orthopaedics & Sports Medicine | THE ORTHOPAEDIC INSTITUTE | |
| OTOLARYNGOLOGY | SOUTH FLORIDA ENT ASSOCIATES | SENTA ENT AND ALLERGY PARTNERS | | |
| RADIOLOGY | rp radiology partners | US Radiology Specialists® Imaging and Interventional Partners | | |

**Fig. 6.** Consolidation of physician practices.

Partners partnership with New York–based Integrated Medical Professionals and Cincinnati-based The Urology Group to form Solaris Health, a management services organization, in 2020.

## POTENTIAL BENEFITS OF PARTNERING WITH PRIVATE EQUITY INVESTMENT

Whether pursuing an initial investment to create a new urology platform or joining an existing platform, there are many potential benefits to taking on private equity capital versus joining a hospital system.

### Equity and Independence

First and foremost, a properly structured private equity agreement gives practice owners a significant equity stake in the business that, as discussed earlier, is a critical element of remaining an independent operator and something hospital systems cannot deliver.

Hand in hand with the financial interest, private equity creates a governance structure that preserves physician authority in areas of critical concern to them and ensures shared decision making between the private equity (PE) firm and physician shareholders. Governance structures vary in scope depending on the issues that are most critical to each practice, but may encompass

issues such as clinical authority, hours, location of practice, the addition of new doctors, and compensation. A good governance model is characterized by inclusivity and collaboration, with a common vision, collective leadership, localized decision making, and a patient-first mindset.

### Liquidity and Future Upside

Many practice owners have a significant portion of their personal net worth tied up in their practice. Partnering with a private equity firm allows them to "take chips off the table" while retaining a significant equity stake that creates a new and potentially larger liquidity opportunity at the time of the private equity firm's sale.

### Addition of Services and Equipment

Urologists in private equity-backed independent group practices can gain access to the capital needed to develop and integrate facility-based services and add new technology in order to provide comprehensive care to patients. Such services may include ambulatory surgery centers, radiation therapy facilities, laboratory, and pharmacy.

### Alleviating Administrative Burdens

Independent physicians work in a much nimbler organization, compared with their counterparts within a health system. By partnering with a larger, privately held entity, physicians can enjoy the benefits of a management services organization that can handle administrative tasks, such as information technology, human resources/benefits, and operations management.

## Network and Operational Enhancements

Practice owners can also gain access to a private equity firm's network, creating opportunities for relationships with suppliers, vendors, and partners they would otherwise not be able to access. Private equity partners can also help improve management processes and financial controls and implement best practices that have proven successful with other providers.

## Legal Protections

Importantly, physicians who retain equity enjoy legal protections not available to physicians whose practices are purchased by hospital ownership groups. They benefit from having a stronger voice in policy, disciplinary, and management decisions. Moreover, once a first private equity deal is struck, the legal protections included as part of that transaction survive and must be honored by subsequent private equity investors, unless physicians agree to renegotiate terms.

## Lowering Payer Costs

Allowing physicians to be successful in private practice environments also drives down costs for payers. According to a 2016 study, the availability of ASCs reduces US health care costs by more than $38 billion per year, driven by lower payments than hospital outpatient department (HOPD) prices for the identical procedure, regardless of market or payer. The study also found that migrating surgical procedures from HOPDs to ASCs could save as much as $55 billion annually.[18]

## EVALUATING AND PREPARING FOR PRIVATE EQUITY INVESTMENT

Although the potential benefits of private equity are evident, it is not a step that should be taken without a great deal of forethought. Taking on any business partner changes the ownership dynamic, and that holds true with private equity. Practice owners should take the time to understand the motivations, perspectives, and methodologies of prospective private equity investors and build consensus with their stakeholders.

## Short- Versus Long-Term Perspective

Physicians need to understand a private equity firm's perspective on time horizon. Private equity firms typically have a 10-year investment time period but may make decisions to accelerate growth or otherwise optimize results to take advantage of market conditions conducive to a successful exit.

Practice owners should ask questions to fully understand the firm's philosophy on investment for long-term sustainable growth rather than short-term gains and weigh it against how they want to run and grow the business. It is critical to understand the firm's target investment horizon and how that might impact investment in the business over time.

## Performance Goals and Incentive Structures

Agreement upfront on whether performance metrics are achievable is a critical piece of a successful private equity partnership. This discussion may need to involve senior professionals in the company whose workload, range of responsibilities, and authority may be impacted by the change. Practice owners also need to have thorough knowledge of how and how frequently performance will be evaluated, what criteria will be used, and the consequences of missing agreed-upon targets.

## Alignment of Stakeholder Interests

Candid discussions to align stakeholder expectations are another critical element of successful private equity partnerships. Physicians should establish a clear understanding with private equity partners of how much they are expected to invest alongside the PE firm. Within the practice itself, it is also important to have transparent conversations about differing concerns and motivations across different classes of physicians, older and younger, partners and nonpartners, to ensure that the agreement is providing fairness and not disenfranchising any group.

## Impact on Quality of Care

Some in the industry have raised concerns about private equity's impact on the quality of care. A good private equity partner should be incentivized to build a sustainable, profitable business with a strong reputation. It is critical to partner with a firm that balances strategies to drive revenue growth and profitability with a commitment to making clinical excellence and patient care paramount.

Once the decision to pursue a private equity investment has been made, it is important to not be a passive participant. The private equity firm will conduct comprehensive due diligence, including legal and regulatory reviews and a detailed analysis of financials and performance metrics. The practice owner must take the same approach, taking a deep dive into the potential investor.

Ask for details on the firm's track record of prior performance in similar investments, what the keys to success were and what influenced their decision to sell. Sometimes failed investments can be even more enlightening. Understanding what went wrong and why, as well as the firm's efforts to save the investment and the lessons they took away from the experience, can tell you a good deal about their strategic approach and character.

Speaking with management teams the private equity team has worked with in the past can provide additional insight into how the firm supports management, their availability to the senior team, the tone and frequency of interaction, and their real commitment and contributions to the company's growth and value creation. Taking a thorough approach to evaluating your private equity partner will help ensure the collaborative and trusting partnership that is essential for success.

No practice owner should take on this burden alone. Trade associations, such as LUGPA, provide forums for private practice leaders to learn about the factors they should consider in deciding whether to partner with private equity.[16] In addition to consulting personal advisors, outside legal and financial counsel from firms specializing in these transactions is advisable, and some practice owners may retain an investment bank to manage interactions with interested firms.

A final consideration independent of firm selection is the timing of a deal process. Seeking investment when revenues are declining is unlikely to result in a positive outcome. Ideally, practice owners should begin a deal process when the practice has had strong and consistent, if not growing, financial results for a year or more. Macro events, such as the pandemic, should also be considered, but if the practice is otherwise strong, they should not be a reason not to pursue a deal.

## UNDERSTANDING THE PRIVATE EQUITY TRANSACTION

To better understand how a private equity transaction with a urology group works, it is important to be familiar with the typical private equity governance model as well as the financial structure of a typical deal. In the following discussion, the authors take a closer look at both.

### Governance

In order for urology practices to pursue a transaction with a private equity group while remaining compliant with state rules and regulations, a new Limited Liability Corporation needs to be created within the corporate structure to which nonclinical, operational assets are transferred; this is commonly known as an MSO.

Through a holding company, physicians retain ownership of the MSO. The private equity partner purchases shares in the holding company from the physicians and claims a fair market value management fee. Typically, the MSO will have a defined role in back office management and will be responsible for nonmedical business and administrative functions, as well as employment of support staff and development of ancillary services. In a healthy relationship, decision making between the MSO and member practices will be collaborative and shared.

Under a standard regional "add-on" platform model, practices are acquired and subsumed by founding practices. By contrast, a national PE-backed urology model creates a balanced system that can be thought of as a *consortium* of regional market-leading partners, governed at a national level by a board of directors that consists of a group CEO, representatives of the private equity partner, and physician leaders. The board is responsible for driving the group's overall growth strategy, reviewing and approving practice merger candidates, and budgeting and making MSO human capital decisions. When new practices join the national group, their existing leadership remains in place, and they work with the national board of directors to identify and realize synergies, both operational and clinical.

### Financial Transaction Structure

Unlike public companies, where profits may be distributed to shareholders in the form of dividends or equity growth, in private physician groups, money earned by the company is distributed back to the doctors on an annual basis, which means that there is no profit for a private equity firm to purchase. The first stage of a private equity transaction therefore involves creating an "artificial profit" by physicians reducing their take-home compensation to create EBITDA (earnings before interest, taxes, depreciation, and amortization), also called an income "rollback." The rollback is calculated based on the spread between market compensation and the current profits of the group.

Once the rollback has been created, the private equity firm purchases it at a multiple. The purchase multiple may vary depending on the specialty (target groups in specialties that have already been somewhat consolidated may command lower multiples), the importance of the target group (whether it is intended to form the nucleus of a new venture, a "platform," or is an "add-on" acquisition to an existing "platform"), and the growth potential of the target group.

The rollback, multiplied by the purchase multiple, becomes the *total enterprise value*. Physicians are beneficiaries of that value, both in the form of immediate cash proceeds and in retained "rollover equity" in the new company. Generally, the private equity firm will expect a meaningful portion of the enterprise value to be rolled into equity in the new enterprise, in order to align incentives for growth between the practice and the private equity company.

For physicians, part of the power of the transaction is the fact that cash proceeds are subject to capital gains tax treatment as opposed to ordinary income. Even assuming that a physician receives no subsequent return on the sale proceeds through further investment and takes no equity stake, the "delta" between capital gains and ordinary income gained by foregoing income and leveraging private equity provides an immediate economic value that might otherwise take the physician a decade to make up.

If one considers that cash proceeds, rather than lying dormant, are reinvested in traditional investment vehicles at a conservative rate of return, the value of the private equity transaction further expands. However, this does not yet factor in an additional important element, the equity stake. By retaining equity in the company, the physician can profit from subsequent transactions, the "second bite".

The benefit of private equity can therefore be longer than 10 years if a reasonable investment return on the cash proceeds is assumed and can be 20 years or more with only 1 successful additional private equity transaction on top of this.

Furthermore, the new revenue streams that can be unlocked by through scale and the private equity partnership, such as ancillary services, big data, and others, create "income repair" that builds back the compensation physicians surrendered in the initial rollback. While in the immediate aftermath of the transaction physician compensation will be lower, these growth initiatives and cost-savings can fill the gap over time.

When one combines the financial impact of upfront cash, the value of investing those proceeds, the value of rollover equity in a subsequent private equity transaction, and income repair, the private equity model can result in income potential that is in excess of traditional independent practice models over time.[19]

## SUMMARY

Throughout the history of urology, clinical excellence has been the foundation and hallmark of successful independent physician practices. By working with the right private equity partner to scale nationally, urologists can maintain high standards of patient care and access the resources needed to invest in growth.

Given the dynamic nature of the sector, it is incumbent on practice leaders to continuously evaluate new opportunities, keeping in mind that maintaining the status quo is a strategic choice not lacking risk. As urology continues to evolve and provides favorable market dynamics to attract investors, urologists should strongly consider the advantages that a private equity partner with aligned interests can bring to the table. These advantages include immediate and future economic value, balanced control, and the resources to compete in an increasingly challenging environment, while maintaining independence.

## DISCLOSURE

The authors are officers of Solaris Health Holdings. Solaris Health Holdings has received private equity investment from Lee Equity Partners.

## REFERENCES

1. Herschman G, Patel A, Kocot L, et al. INSIGHT: health-care consolidation strong in 2019—expect even stronger 2020. Bloomberg Law. 2020. Available at: https://news.bloomberglaw.com/health-law-and-business/insight-health-care-consolidation-strong-in-2019-expect-even-stronger-2020. Accessed November 5, 2020.
2. Daly R. Number of Medicare ACOs stays flat, but risk-taking increases. HFMA.org. 2020. Available at: https://www.hfma.org/topics/news/2020/01/number-of-medicare-acos-stays-flat-but-risk-taking-increases.html. Accessed November 5, 2020.
3. Suthrum P. Physician practice consolidation: it's only just begun. STATnews.com. 2020. Available at: https://www.statnews.com/2020/02/27/physician-practice-consolidation-its-only-just-begun/. Accessed November 5, 2020.
4. UnitedHealth's optum to acquire surgical care affiliates for $2.3 billion. Modern healthcare. 2017. Available at: https://www.modernhealthcare.com/article/20170109/NEWS/170109936/unitedhealth-s-optum-to-acquire-surgical-care-affiliates-for-2-3-billion. Accessed November 5, 2020.

5. The state of the urology workforce and practice in the United States 2019. American Urological Association. 2020. Available at: https://www.auanet.org/documents/research/census/2019%20The%20State%20of%20the%20Urology%20Workforce%20Census%20Book.pdf. Accessed November 5, 2020.

6. List of largest urology practices in U.S. Brighter health network. 2019. Available at: https://www.bhnco.com/Resources/largest-urology-practices-in-unitedstates.html. Accessed November 5, 2020.

7. Martin K. Medscape urologist compensation report 2020. Medscape. 2020. https://www.medscape.com/slideshow/2020-compensation-urologist-6012749. Accessed November 5, 2020.

8. Katz M. Private equity funds raise nearly $600 billion in 2019. Chief investment officer. 2020. Available at: https://www.ai-cio.com/news/private-equity-funds-raise-nearly-600-billion-2019/. Accessed November 5, 2020.

9. Rooney K. Private equity's record $1.5 trillion cash pile comes with a new set of challenges. CNBC.com. 2020. Available at: https://www.cnbc.com/2020/01/03/private-equitys-record-cash-pile-comes-with-a-new-set-of-challenges.html. Accessed November 5, 2020.

10. MacArthur H, Lerner J. Public vs. private equity returns: is PE losing its advantage? Bain & company. 2020. Available at: https://www.bain.com/insights/public-vs-private-markets-global-private-equity-report-2020/. Accessed November 5, 2020.

11. Cordeiro N, Hanson B, Sam J. US PE middle market report. PitchBook. 2017. Available at: https://www.acg.org/sites/files/PitchBook_2Q_2017_US_PE_Middle_Market_Report_0.pdf. Accessed November 5, 2020.

12. Davis SG, Carmean Z. US PE middle market report, Q1 2020. PitchBook. 2020. Available at: https://pitchbook.com/news/reports/q1-2020-us-pe-middle-market-report. Accessed November 5, 2020.

13. Global healthcare private equity and corporate M&A Report 2020. Bain & Company. 2020. Available at: https://www.bain.com/globalassets/noindex/2020/bain_report_global_healthcare_private_equity_and_corporate_ma_report_2020.pdf. Accessed November 5, 2020.

14. Saenz A. How private equity can improve the health of healthcare. EY. 2019. Available at: https://www.ey.com/en_us/private-equity/how-private-equity-can-improve-the-health-of-healthcare. Accessed November 5, 2020.

15. Caldwell HM. Health organizations find themselves in the eye of a perfect storm. EY. 2020. Available at: https://www.ey.com/en_us/ccb/health-mergers-acquisitions. Accessed November 5, 2020.

16. Zhu J, Hua L, Polsky D. Private equity acquisitions of physician medical groups across specialties, 2013-2016. JAMA. 2020. Available at: https://jamanetwork.com/journals/jama/article-abstract/2761076. Accessed November 5, 2020.

17. Palamara K, Major E, Aprill R. Private practice consolidation opportunity in the fragmented urology specialty. Provident. 2017. Available at: https://www.providenthp.com/wp-content/uploads/2020/03/Private-Practice-Consolidation-Opportunity-in-the-Fragmented-Urology-Specialty.pdf. Accessed November 5, 2020.

18. Commercial insurance cost savings in ambulatory surgery centers. Healthcare Bluebook, ambulatory surgery center association, HealthSmart. Available at: https://www.ascassociation.org/HigherLogic/System/DownloadDocumentFile.ashx?DocumentFileKey=829b1dd6-0b5d-9686-e57c-3e2ed4ab42ca&forceDialog=0. Accessed November 5, 2020.

19. Zhu J, Hua L, Polsky D. Private Equity Acquisitions of Physician Medical Groups Across Specialties, 2013-2016. JAMA. Available at: https://jamanetwork.com/journals/jama/article-abstract/2761076. Published February 18, 2020. Accessed November 5, 2020.

# Clinical Research 2021

Evan R. Goldfischer, MD, MBA, CPE, CPI

## KEYWORDS

- Clinical research • Clinical trials • Regulation • Protocol

## KEY POINTS

- Clinical research is of great benefit to patients and rewarding to clinicians.
- Clinical research in the United States is highly regulated.
- There are significant penalties for violating protocols.
- Clinical research requires a good infrastructure in each practice.

## MANAGING A RESEARCH PROGRAM IN 2021
### Why Do It and What Are Benefits of Doing It?

During residency and fellowship programs, most urologists have an opportunity for clinical and/or basic science research. When choosing private practice, however, many urologists believe this opportunity would be lost. Doing research in private practice is extremely rewarding and uses skills not used routinely in the course of clinical practice. It is an opportunity to be on the cutting edge of urology treatment and to use pharmaceutical agents before they are approved by the Food and Drug Administration (FDA). Common research trials in recent years have included studies of drugs and devices for benign prostatic hyperplasia, erectile dysfunction, stress urinary continence, bladder cancer, prostate cancer, kidney cancer, overactive bladder, and other conditions. It is an opportunity to offer patients who have failed traditional therapy a new option, and it can help retain patients who often might have to travel a great distance to an academic medical center to have access to these agents. In addition, it can be rewarding and enjoyable for clinicians when a drug ultimately is approved, and the urologists concerned then are experts among their peers because they have been using a drug/device for several years prior to FDA approval. It also can be a source of revenue for the practice, but financial gain should not be a reason for establishing a clinical research program in private practice. In summary, a clinical research program directly benefits patients by giving them access to drugs and devices when the patients have failed or cannot tolerate traditional therapy; a clinical research program allows a practice to retain patients instead of referring them to an academic medical center that might require the patients to travel a great distance; it can be a source of revenue; and it allows a urologist to become a credible expert on a new treatment by having used the therapy prior to FDA approval.

### The Research Landscape in 2021

The research landscape has changed dramatically over the past decade. The clinical trials in urology are focused more on oncology than on other areas, and these trials often require recruitment of patients with very specific characteristics, making it difficult to have high-volume recruitment for any single trial. The devices also are more sophisticated and require specific inclusion criteria. In addition, there has been significant consolidation in the contract research organization (CRO) business, so relationships with the current CROs are important. Finally, sponsors, institutional review boards (IRBs), and the FDA have been exercising more oversight, so it is important that every research site be prepared for a time-consuming audit.

### Practice Support

One physician cannot drive a successful research program. Research must be an initiative that the entire practice supports, because it requires all of the providers to understand the trials and to participate in recruitment. The primary investigator (PI) for the trial must be given time during the day

Urology Division, Premier Medical Group, New York Medical College
E-mail address: egoldfischer@premiermedicalhv.com

Urol Clin N Am 48 (2021) 245–250
https://doi.org/10.1016/j.ucl.2021.01.005

urologic.theclinics.com

to perform the clinical visits, meet with research staff, and meet with the clinical monitors. If the practice compensates its providers on a productivity model, then the PI must be compensated appropriately.

## Types of Clinical Trials

Phase I trials often require an inpatient research facility and are the most difficult trials to conduct because a drug is being tested in a small group of humans, often for the first time, and the full range of side effects is unknown. In phase I trials, the subjects and the researchers know the drug and the dosage that they are receiving, and the dose usually is escalated until such time as the subjects experience significant side effects.

In phase II trials, the experimental drug or treatment is given to a larger group of people at a specified dose or several doses to test its efficacy and monitor side effects. Sometimes, if the drug is being tested in a rare disease state that has limited opportunity for recruitment, a phase II trial actually can lead to FDA approval in certain circumstances.

Phase III trials are the most common trials conducted in a private practice clinical research program. These usually are double-blind trials conducted across many sites in large numbers of patients at specified doses to truly measure efficacy and safety of a new drug.

Phase IV trials are postmarketing studies conducted after a drug has been approved for treatment by the FDA and provide additional information about a drug's risks and benefits.[1]

These are the accepted 4 phases of clinical trials, but the studies themselves can be classified by category:

Treatment research—involves drugs, devices, or new therapies to effect a cure for a disease state

Prevention research—looks for therapies to prevent disorders from developing or recurring

Diagnostic research—looks for new ways to identify a disorder or condition

Screening research—finds the best ways to identify a disorder or condition

Quality of life research—seeks to find ways to improve the quality of life for patients with chronic conditions

Genetic studies—seek to understand how genes and disorders are related. These studies are becoming much more common, particularly in oncology.

Epidemiologic studies—try to identify patterns and causes of disease[2]

Note that some clinical trials are designed to gather a substantial amount of data and can overlap in several of these categories, particularly in oncology.

## Clinical Research Organizations

Many trial sponsors do not have the resources to conduct a clinical trial, so they hire professional CROs to recruit sites, conduct the trials, and in some cases analyze the data. A CRO may provide services, such as biopharmaceutical development, biologic assay development, commercialization, preclinical research, clinical research, clinical trials management, and pharmacovigilance.

## Staffing

### Principal investigator/medical director

Once a practice decides to embark on a clinical research program, it needs to hire dedicated staff who are assigned exclusively to the program. The PI, who usually serves as the medical director for the program, needs to have time carved out of the normal work week to oversee the program, conduct patient visits, review results, and monitor patient compliance and side effects. The FDA regards the PI as the individual who is responsible for the conduct of the trial at the study site, and, although the PI may delegate responsibilities, ultimately the PI is responsible for everything that happens at the site.

### Subinvestigators

In a large practice, the PI has other clinical responsibilities, so other physicians and advanced practice providers are able to serve as subinvestigators to ensure compliance with the research protocol and to help recruit patients into the trials.

### Lead clinical coordinator

The lead clinical coordinator leads the research team on a day-to-day basis. It helps, greatly, if this person is a registered nurse or licensed practical nurse so that they have the skills to draw blood, start intravenous lines, administer medications, and perform electrocardiograms and other clinical tasks. They should be experienced, to understand the importance of meticulous documentation and how to handle an FDA audit. This individual is responsible for training the other coordinators and should have a reasonable knowledge of reviewing and negotiating research budgets. In short, this person is the key member of the team.

### Clinical coordinator

Clinical coordinators are delegated tasks by the PI and, like the lead coordinator, should be dedicated to research and not have other responsibilities in the practice. They need to have good clinical skills and great rapport with patients because some of the research visits can be quite long. An experienced coordinator, depending on the complexity of the trial, typically can handle 1 to 2 trials in the active recruiting phase, 1 to 2 trials in the clinical visit stage, and 2 to 3 trials in the follow-up stage after most of the visits have been completed.[3]

## Resources

### Data and information technology support

Although many sponsors of clinical research trials provide an advertising budget to recruit patients from outside the practice, most patients who are enrolled into trials are patients of the practice, so maintaining a good database and being able to use analytical tools to scan the electronic medical record system are extremely important. It is important for a site to take a clinical trial only if it has the staffing and resources to conduct the trial properly. Also, because it is expensive for a sponsor to initiate a site, if a site performs poorly by having multiple protocol violations during monitoring visits or fails to meet its recruitment goals, the site could be blacklisted and not given any more trials in the future by the sponsor or CRO.

### Standard operating procedures

Every research site should have a handbook of standard operating procedures (SOPs) for all tasks that could be required of site personnel. Every member of the team should sign the book, indicating that they have read it and agree to comply with the SOPs. It should be updated on a regular basis. Although SOP binders are available for purchase, it is better if they are developed in house and reflect the actual practices of the site.

## Regulatory and Compliance

### Form 1572

FDA Form 1572 as well as a financial disclosure form should be completed by all individuals at the research stie for each clinical trial. The form is published by the FDA and should be updated on an annual basis or if circumstances change where a site member has a significant financial or other conflict in performing the trials.[4]

### Good Clinical Practice

Good Clinical Practice (GCP) is an international ethical and scientific quality standard for the design, conduct, performance, monitoring, auditing, recording, analyses, and reporting of clinical trials. It also serves to protect the rights, integrity, and confidentiality of trial subjects. Most sponsors of clinical trials require site personal to be GCP certified and the certification to be updated on a regular basis. GCP courses are available online.[5]

### Code of Federal Regulations

The FDA, having been given Congressional authority, creates the rules and regulations for conducting clinical research. These regulations, although technically not laws, have the force of law and are codified in the Code of Federal Regulations (CFR), and there are serious penalties for not following them, including being banned from conducting clinical research.[6]

### Institutional review board

An IRB is an administrative body established to protect the rights and welfare of human research subjects recruited to participate in research activities. Most academic institutions that conduct clinical research have their own IRBs, whereas clinical research conducted at private practice sites often uses a nationally recognized central IRB. The members of an IRB usually include clinicians, researchers, clergy, ethicists, and members from the community at large. The job of the IRB is not to write or rewrite a protocol but to protect the rights and welfare of all patients enrolled in the trials, to monitor the studies for adverse events (AEs) and serious adverse events (SAEs), and to review and approve all amendments to the protocols. Members are obligated to recuse themselves if they have a conflict of interest.[7]

## Adverse Events

An AE is any untoward medical occurrence in a patient or clinical investigation subject administered a pharmaceutical product and that does not necessarily have a causal relationship with this treatment (**Box 1**).[8] This is a broad definition and is designed to capture anything that a patient reports as different while participating in a clinical trial. The sponsor provides a timeline for the reporting of AEs and requires the PI to decide if the AE is related to the treatment that the patient is receiving in the trial. The AEs are reported to the IRB, and the IRB has the power to halt or to terminate the trial in order to protect the patients enrolled in the trial. AEs are graded (see **Box 1**).

### Serious Adverse Events

An SAE is an AE that results in death, a life-threatening experience, inpatient hospitalization, a persistent or significant disability or incapacity, or a congenital anomaly or birth defect.[9] An SAE usually must be reported to the sponsor and IRB

---

**Box 1**
**Grading of adverse events**

Grade 1: mild or minimal symptoms. Intervention rarely is indicated.

Grade 2: moderate symptoms. Minimal or noninvasive intervention is required.

Grade 3: severe symptoms requiring medical intervention, but not life threatening

Grade 4: life threatening event requiring urgent care

Grade 5: death

---

within 24 hours of the event occurring. Failure to do so could result in the closing of the research site. Ultimately, it is the decision of the PI at the site to decide if an SAE has occurred and to determine the causality to the trial.

## Monitoring Visits

During the conduct of the trial, the sponsor or CRO managing the trial conducts regular visits to the site to ensure compliance with the protocol.[10] There usually is a visit to the site before site selection, a start-up visit to review the protocol, a visit after the first subject is enrolled, regular visits during the trial, and then at least 1 close-out visit. It is important that the study coordinator in charge of the trial be available during these visits to the study monitor as well as the lead coordinator. The monitor usually wants to meet with the PI to discuss the findings of the visit and usually sends a formal letter discussing any deficiencies found during the visit, which must be reviewed and corrected, if possible. It is important that the monitor finish the visit feeling that the PI truly is involved in supervising the trial and is aware of the enrolled subjects, has conducted the visits, and has reported any AEs.

## Budget Development and Accounting

Research can be a profit center for the practice, but money should not be the motivating factor to establish a clinical research program. Many programs believe they are profitable when in fact they are losing money. It is important to negotiate a start-up fee from the sponsor that covers the fixed costs of the trial and to negotiate an archiving fee when the trial is done, because most sponsors want the records stored on site for at least 6 months and then off site in perpetuity. When calculating budgets, be sure to include rent; utilities; depreciation on equipment, such as refrigerated centrifuges; and costs of performing

examinations, blood draws, and other diagnostic tests, including radiologic studies. Shipping containers, dry ice, wet ice, and packing materials also should be budget line items. In short, if a site is not attentive to every detail in the study and the time required from each member of the research team, the trial could result in a substantial financial loss even if enrollment was good.

## Sources of Clinical Trials

### Industry

Industry-sponsored trials are one of the most common sources of clinical trials and typically have the best budgets because the sponsor intends to sell the drug or device for a profit after receiving FDA approval.[11] Often, the trials are managed by CROs, and the sponsors review their databases to see which sites have performed well in past trials. It is important for a site to decline a trial if they do not have the resources or patient population that has been requested. Advertising well yields some new patients but advertising cannot be relied on predominantly to fill the trial slots. Budget negotiations take place with the CRO or the industry sponsor directly, who has a record of what the site was paid in the past. If costs have increased or the trial is more complex and requires more resources, a case usually can be made for an increased budget, especially if the site has performed well in the past. Medical science liaisons who visit the practice often are knowledgeable about upcoming clinical trials for their company and can recommend sites.

### Cooperative groups

Cooperative groups include the Society of Urologic Oncology Clinical Trials Consortium, the Southwest Oncology Group, the Radiation Therapy Oncology Group, the Eastern Cooperative Oncology Group, the Comprehensive Unit-based Safety Program, and others. The National Cancer Institute funds these groups to study adult cancers. Membership usually is required to participate in the trials, and most of the members are academic centers. The budgets for these trials are not lucrative and often barely cover costs. The trials, however, usually are well designed, and participation in them is considered prestigious.

### Investigator-initiated trials

Most pharmaceutical companies encourage investigator-initiated trials (IITs). The process to approval can be laborious, and the budgets usually are limited. Conducting an IIT can be rewarding but requires a lot of resources from the site, which essentially serves as its own CRO and must follow GCP and FDA regulations. Only sites that have an experienced PI with experienced staff should undertake IITs.

### Academic center

If a private practice site has a good relationship with the local academic medical center, then the academic center may reach out to the private site to help with patient recruitment because private groups often see a higher volume of patients. These trials usually are funded by industry or federal grants, so the budgets are limited but can provide an opportunity for patients to have access to a novel treatment.

## Subject Recruitment

Site databases are the best way to recruit subjects for clinical trials. It is good practice to keep a log of all patients who are screened for a particular disease state, because they may screen fail for a specific trial but might meet criteria for another trial.[12] Also, sometimes patients who complete a trial and have had a good experience may be willing to participate in future trials. Using the electronic medical record, it also is possible to search for patients with specific conditions who might consider enrolling in a trial.

Most sponsors provide IRB-approved signs that can be placed in waiting rooms advertising for a specific trial. Radio, television, and newspaper advertisements also can be helpful. Clinical research trials also can be advertised on a practice Web site.

Staff members, such as medical assistants and nurses who interact with patients, can suggest to patients that they speak with the doctor about a clinical trial. Urodynamics nurses often know if a patient is a candidate for a clinical incontinence trial and can discuss the options with the patient.

Patient support groups for various disease states, including prostate cancer, bladder cancer, interstitial cystitis, and incontinence, should be notified about new clinical trials and opportunities for patients who have failed traditional therapies.

It is important to let the referring physicians know that about the research and, although a practice may not have an IRB-approved recruitment letter for every trial, it certainly is acceptable to let referring physicians know that a practice does clinical research and the broad disease characteristics of the ongoing trials. Patients in clinical trials also may refer friends to the site.

## Audits

Audits can be conducted by the sponsor, the CRO, the IRB, or the FDA.[13] Sometimes the audit is for a specific cause, if a deficiency is suspected, and sometimes it is a random audit, particularly if a site is high enrolling in a clinical trial. An FDA audit is a serious and time-consuming affair, so most sponsors require that if a site is served notice by the FDA of an impending audit, the site must contact the sponsor so that they can send in a team to help the site prepare for the FDA visit. Depending on the number of visits and length of the clinical trial, an FDA audit can last days, weeks, or even months, so the entire research team should be available while the FDA is on site.

According to the FDA, the "FDA conducts clinical investigator inspections to determine if the clinical investigators are conducting clinical studies in compliance with applicable statutory and regulatory requirements. Clinical investigators who conduct FDA-regulated clinical investigations are required to permit FDA investigators to access, copy, and verify any records or reports made by the clinical investigator with regard to, among other records, the disposition of the investigational product and subjects' case histories. See 21 CFR 312.68 and 812.145. The FDA investigator typically performs this oversight function through on-site inspections designed to document how the study was actually conducted at the clinical investigator's site. For investigational drug studies, clinical investigators must retain study records for a period of two years following the date a marketing application is approved for the drug for the indication for which it is being investigated; or, if no application is to be filed or if the application is not approved for such indication, until two years after the investigation is discontinued and FDA is notified. See 21 CFR 312.62(c)."

There are several outcomes that can result from an FDA audit. The best action is no deficiencies as the inspector finds that the site was in total compliance. The next level is a written 483 form. The 483 describes any inspectional observations that, in the opinion of the FDA investigator conducting the inspection, represent deviations from applicable statutes and regulations. A FDA Form 483 usually results when there are protocol violations, documentation deficiencies, informed consent issues, or accountability of the investigational product. The FDA also can issue a warning letter to the site if more significant violations are found, and, finally, the FDA can close a research site and bar the investigator and subinvestigators from doing research in the future.

## DISCLOSURES

The author has nothing to disclose.

## REFERENCES

1. Available at: https://www.nccn.org/patients/resources/clinical_trials/phases.aspx.

2. Available at: https://www.fda.gov/patients/clinical-trials-what-patients-need-know/what-are-different-types-clinical-research.

3. Available at: https://www.partners.org/Assets/Documents/Medical-Research/Clinical-Research/Study-Staff-Information-Sheet.pdf.

4. Available at: https://www.cancer.gov/publications/dictionaries/cancer-terms/def/form-fda-1572-statement-of-investigator.

5. Available at: https://www.fda.gov/files/medical%20devices/published/Presentation–Good-Clinical-Practice-101–An-Introduction-%28PDF-Version%29.pdf.

6. Available at: https://www.hhs.gov/ohrp/sites/default/files/ohrp/policy/ohrpregulations.pdf.

7. Available at: https://www.fda.gov/regulatory-information/search-fda-guidance-documents/institutional-review-boards-frequently-asked-questions.

8. Available at: https://dipg.org/dipg-research/clinical-trials-for-dipg/side-effects/.

9. Available at: https://www.ackc.org/common-terminology-criteria-for-adverse-events/.

10. Available at: https://www.fda.gov/media/116754/download.

11. Available at: https://clinicaltrials.gov/ct2/resources.

12. Available at: https://www.pharmavoice.com/article/clinical-trial-recruitment-0615/.

13. Available at: https://www.fda.gov/media/75185/download.

# Health Policy and Advocacy

Thomas H. Rechtschaffen, MD[a],*, Deepak A. Kapoor, MD[b,1]

**KEYWORDS**

- Advocacy • Health policy • Physician leadership

**KEY POINTS**

- Engagement in health policy and advocacy is critical to the future of the practice of medicine.
- The 3 major urologic organizations (American Urological Association, American Association of Clinical Urologists, and Large Urology Group Practice Association) evolved different pathways to engage the national and state legislative and policy apparatus.
- Urology engagement has resulted in significant impact on the practice of medicine on both state and federal levels from both legislative and regulatory perspectives.
- The importance of individual contributions from both time and money to political efforts cannot be overstated.
- Increasing diversity among those involved in leadership and advocacy is needed to amplify urologists' voice over the coming years.

## PHYSICIAN ADVOCACY IN HEALTH POLICY—HOW? WHY NOW? AND WHY ME?

The scope of interest of those pursuing medical careers has greatly changed—30 years ago, other than the occasional associated PhD, medical students an physicians rarely pursued degrees beyond an MD. Physicians now commonly pursue additional studies outside of their medical training, whether it be degrees in law, business, hospital administration, or public health—the Association of American Medical Colleges reports that from 2006 to 2014, the number of physicians graduating from medical school with dual degrees increased by more than 50%,[1] amplifying the importance of expanded expertise to aspects other than direct patient care. The ability for practicing urologists to enter the arena of health policy and advocacy has expanded as their knowledge base and experience has increased; although it may not always seem the case, the input of practicing physicians of a variety of backgrounds is actively sought by legislators and regulatory agencies because this input is essential for patients' access to the level of care that current knowledge and technologies.

As with most life endeavors, the most daunting step in political engagement is the first one. Many practicing urologists may feel unqualified to comment on health policy, may feel uncomfortable engaging with the political apparatus, and have very real concerns about whether this engagement can produce tangible results. Perhaps most importantly, even interested physicians struggle find time to be engaged effectively in this arena with commitments to amass relative value unit expectations, research activities, Centers for Medicare & Medicaid Services (CME) requirements and other certification burdens, and time for family life and personal pursuits. Given these constraints, typically, there is a perceived need or threat that overcomes these obstacles to engagement and overcomes inertia. Whether it be the historical threat to lithotripsy partnerships defeated by the American Lithotripsy Society,[2] the need to protect dedicated armed forces

[a] Integrated Medical Professionals, PLLC, Farmingdale, NY, USA; [b] Icahn School of Medicine at Mount Sinai, New York, NY, USA
[1] Present address: 340 Broadhollow Road, Farmingdale, NY 11735.
* Corresponding author. 21 Ridgecrest East, Scarsdale, NY 10583.
*E-mail address:* trechtschaffen@imppllc.com

Urol Clin N Am 48 (2021) 251–258
https://doi.org/10.1016/j.ucl.2021.01.007

personnel from wartime injuries,[3] challenges to the ability to develop integrated care models,[4] or unelected regulatory bodies making medical determinations potentially depriving patients of lifesaving diagnostic testing,[5–7] to name but a few, many physicians involved in health policy were galvanized by a specific event. In addition to responding to events, such as these, organized urology societies provide regular input to legislative and regulatory bodies via engagement through commentary on the Medicare Physician Fee Schedule and Outpatient Prospective Payment System annual rules. Consequently, there is an organized infrastructure in place for physicians who become motivated to engage for whatever reason.

That said, despite potential difficulties in becoming part of the process, it is the overwhelming experience of those who engage in policy and advocacy that the benefits to engagement have far outweighed the challenges in becoming engaged. Career satisfaction improves with involvement, the likelihood of burnout decreases, and it helps develop strong physician leadership skills. Physician leaders explain complex medical issues to lay individuals in government that typically view policy issues through a political lens— understanding the real-world impact and potential unintended consequences of their actions is vital to the job performance of legislative and regulatory agencies. Legislators, particularly in the US House of Representatives, welcome the input of physicians practicing in their communities to a degree that is surprising to those starting in the advocacy process. Eventually, as relationships develop, these leaders view physicians that engage with them not only as advocates but also as a resource and actively seek input pending legislation and regulations, which can have profound effects on a urologist's ability to practice. The corollary to this also is true—physician leaders can translate complex legislative and regulatory processes to fellow physicians to help colleagues navigate what for many can be bewildering and rapid changes to their practice.

## LEGISLATION VERSUS REGULATION— ADVOCACY BY SPECIALTY SOCIETIES

For many years, the urologic community met for the Joint Advocacy Conference met every spring in Washington, DC. This meeting, comanaged by the American Association of Clinical Urologists (AACU) and the American Urological Association (AUA), included briefings on the health policy priorities of organized urology and culminated with visits to Capitol Hill to engage with congressional leaders. And although the 2 groups separated after 2017, each has continued its own meeting annually. The Large Urology Group Practice Association (LUGPA) adopts a somewhat different strategy, one of highly targeted engagement through focused bipartisan political giving to members of the key committees of jurisdiction, as discussed previously. Thus, rather than a single large gathering of physicians, the LUGPA typically conducts small group meetings every 6 weeks to 8 weeks. Regardless of approach, this immersion into how health policy affects the day-to-day practice of medicine and the power of participation in advocacy is unique and impactful. Regrettably, the recent public health emergency has severely curtailed these interactions, and, although they continue virtually, clearly are less impactful that the face-to-face interactions previously employed.

Despite the existence of highly organized policy and advocacy infrastructures, it is remarkable that the spectrum of the activities available within the AUA, AACU, and LUGPA still is a surprise to many urologists. Part of this is a consequence of medical training—although it is clearly a first responsibility to understand the disease processes of the genitourinary tract and how to treat them with a combination of medication, surgery, and lifestyle modification strategies, there is no time dedicated within residency education requirements to health policy. Those who engage in policy feel this is a tremendous shortcoming because it does no one any good to learn a skill that cannot be utilized due to legislative or regulatory fiat. Happily, this is changing. The AUA has increased its focus on programs through to deliver grand rounds lectures on these very subjects, exposing the newest in the ranks to health policy. The AUA also offers career development programs, which include its leadership program for urologists in the first decade of practice, the Holtgrewe Fellowship for residents and fellows, and the Gallagher Health Policy Scholarship for those in practice. Health policy activities on the section level and committees on the national level also are powerful ways to contribute time and energy. The legislative affairs committee within the Public Policy Council assembles the AUA legislative priorities are released by the AUA board every year based on the general membership's preferences.

The LUGPA Forward program seeks to engage younger practitioners, creating a subgroup of physicians who recently have completed residency. Representatives from this group participate in LUGPA's sophisticated political affairs and health policy apparatus. These committees rely heavily on the development of long-term relationships by highly experienced physician leaders. This system creates in effect an apprenticeship program, where engaged younger physicians participate in LUGPA events on a regular basis, eventually conducting them on their own. This has enabled LUGPA, despite being a relatively fledgling organization, to develop and maintain a robust advocacy infrastructure.

The AACU's health policy apparatus focuses on state advocacy through the state society network. This is an essential component to policy work because many regulations and laws are promulgated on the state level—given the degree of scrutiny on every action on the federal level, actions on the state level that potentially are impactful on the practice of medicine can happen quickly and without much oversight. By monitoring state activity, the AACU successfully has triggered efforts to combat adverse legislation in several states, often engaging other specialty societies and stakeholders. In addition, AACU is fully engaged with AUA and LUGPA on federal issues.

Communication between specialty societies in urology continues to improve. Physician leaders in policy and advocacy understand that, although different groups may have different constituencies and priorities, the need for urology as a specialty to speak with single voice never has been greater. The health policy apparatus on both physician and staff levels for the AUA, AACU, and LUGPA communicate regularly and have scheduled meetings no less than monthly. Through these efforts, intersociety communication and collaboration are at their highest levels, greatly benefitting the specialty as a whole.

At present, skills needed to become effective advocates for patients are not part of the residency curriculum; certainly, there is a concerted effort to enhance awareness to the need for these efforts early in urologists' careers.

## UROTRAUMA BILL—RELATIONSHIPS BUILT AND LESSONS LEARNED

The wars of this century in the Middle East have seen increased use of improvised explosive devices, which explode typically from below a solider who may be riding in a vehicle. This can result in injuries that more often cause lower extremity and pelvic damage—this is in contrast to previous conflicts, when projectiles were used that were more likely to cause injuries to the head or torso and upper extremities.[3]

As the principal providers of care to the genitourinary tract, management of these injuries falls in large part to urologists; as such, many other practitioners simply were unaware of the magnitude of this problem. Consequently, there was no. Unlike programs already in existence for other organ systems (such as traumatic brain injury), there was no organized effort to evaluate the impact of and optimize treatment of these novel pelvic injuries. As such, it fell to the urologic community to advocate for men and women of the armed forces who risk their lives.

This resulted in the development of the Urotrauma bill, which directed the Department of Defense to establish an entity devoted to care for military personnel who suffer injuries to the urinary tract in combat.[8] This effort diverged from prior policy work in that rather than seeking to thwart adverse legislation and rulemaking, The Urotrauma legislation was a proactive piece of legislation. Any piece of legislation, regardless of how noble in purpose and nominal in cost, is extremely difficult to pass.

This legislation provided important learnings on the mechanics of promulgating legislation. Seeking the appropriate sponsors and cosponsors, having bipartisan champions in both the House and the Senate, identifying the proper committees through which to introduce the bill, developing budgetary offsets, and navigating the legislative schedule were merely some of the challenges that needed to be overcome.

The cynicism physicians feel for lawmakers is reciprocated to a certain degree, because legislators are fearful of angering one set of constituents when they act in favor of another; in addition, any ask that has an impact on budgets have a much harder hill to climb to become law. Consequently, although the budgetary ask was a mere $4 million and no legislator was opposed, this bill required substantial effort over several years to be passed. Through these efforts, that resulted in no economic gain to urologists but completely focused on the nation's wounded warriors, the efforts to pass this legislation built connections with Senate and House members and changed the optics by which the specialty is viewed. The relationships on the Hill built on this moral and unselfish ask have served the specialty well for all of the years since then. Bills often take several sessions of congress to pass, and the party in control of the agendas and the committees may flip multiple times during that time. Having broad support from both parties ensured that this legislation proposal would be reintroduced with each new session. With persistence over several years by dedicated urologists and congressional sponsors, aided by joint advocacy by the AUA, AACU, and LUGPA, the Urotrauma bill language eventually was included in the National Defense Authorization Act of 2014 and signed into law.

## THE US PREVENTIVE SERVICES TASK FORCE AND PROSTATE-SPECIFIC ANTIGEN: AN EXAMPLE OF MULTIDISCIPLINARY ADVOCACY

As most urologists are aware, in 2012, the US Preventive Services Task Force (USPSTF) issued a grade D recommendation on the use of serum prostate-specific antigen (PSA) as a screening tool for the early detection of prostate cancer.[5] Most urologists also are aware that this recommendation was updated to a grade C recommendation, which emphasizes shared decision making; however, most are aware of neither the complexities regarding the USPSTF recommendations nor the urology community's sustained response. This action represents a comprehensive case study on the power and importance of physician leadership and advocacy.

To understand the complexities that arose with advocacy around the USPSTF PSA recommendations, it is necessary to understand the history of the USPSTF specifically and of Medicare preventive services in general. When Medicare was signed into law in 1966 by President Lyndon B. Johnson, it was designed to cover acute care; preventive services (eg, checking blood pressure in otherwise healthy individuals) were not covered benefits. Despite the ongoing and increased recognition of the value of such services in enhancing health, the CMS as a regulatory agency did not have authority to add benefits specified under statute—any alterations of Medicare benefits had to come from congressional legislative action. To accomplish this, by 1980 more than 350 bills were introduced to cover these types of services.[9]

To help provide guidance on these services, in 1984 the USPSTF was created with representation from the disciplines of internal medicine, family medicine, pediatrics, behavioral health, obstetrics-gynecology, and nursing. At the time of formation, the USPSTF served as a purely advisory entity; there was no obligation for any regulatory agency, Congress, or provider to follow their guidance. As such, the USPSTF was not required to comply with 2 key federal oversight acts, the Federal Advisory Committee Act and the Administrative Procedure Act. As an advisory body with no binding economic authority, it was exempt from rules, including providing a public comment period to its recommendation, transparency of its process of appointing members, release of methodology and communications on how the members reached their conclusions, and exemption from the freedom of information act, among others. Of particular consternation to specialty societies is that not only is there no representation of

specialists directly responsible for providing the services being reviewed but also there is no requirement for the USPSTF to consult content specific experts when considering preventive care.

Even with the creation of the USPSTF, addition of preventive services proved challenging—by 1993, only 4 of 44 services recommended by the USPSTF for the elderly were covered by Medicare.[9] The problem of benefits lagging progress in preventive services was addressed more formally in 2008 with the passage of the Medicare Improvements for Patients and Providers Act (MIPPA).[10] Although preventive services went through a process of National Coverage Determinations, the views of the USPSTF were given substantial credence—CMS was granted the independent authority to add services deemed reasonable and necessary provided they received an A or B recommendation from the USPSTF. Although MIPPA did not allow for denial of services based on USPSTF recommendations, for the first and only time in US history, an advisory board not subject to federal oversight was granted the authority to make recommendations that result in changes to payment policy.

With the passage of the Patient Protection and Affordable Care Act of 2010 (ACA), colloquially known as Obamacare, the authority of the USPSTF was greatly expanded.[11] The CMS were mandated to cover services with a USPSTF grade A or grade B recommendation; ominously, the authority to deny services with a grade D recommendation was created and, by inference, the CMS were granted the authority to deny services simply if the USPSTF elected to provide a recommendation. As such, the authority to cover or deny services was placed solely in the hands of an agency completely outside the federal regulatory oversight process.

This history set the stage for the USPSTF recommendations regarding prostate cancer screening. To be clear, 2012 was not the first time that the USPSTF had evaluated PSA-based prostate cancer screening. In its prior reviews, the USPST had issued I recommendations, meaning that there was insufficient category I data to evaluate the efficacy of the test.[12] That changed in 2012 with the issuance of a grade D recommendation, which went so far as to say the harms of a simple blood test outweighed any potential benefits.[5] This was a 1-size-fits-all policy and did not consider the impact of family history, environmental toxin exposure, or race on prostate cancer risk—all clearly egregious oversights.

The response of the urologic community to the USPSTF grade D recommendation was swift, varying from serious concerns to outright condemnation. As a baseline, the science surrounding PSA testing underwent an expert-based review. The AUA published updated prostate cancer screening guidelines[9] that emphasized shared decision making; similar efforts were endorsed by the LUGPA and the AACU. Simultaneously, there was broad outreach to the primary care community, both informal and formal, on the importance of PSA testing, particularly in high-risk populations. Perhaps most importantly was engagement with patient advocacy groups, both broad based and representing specific constituencies (ie, veterans exposed to Agent Orange and the African American community).

These foundational advocacy efforts proved critical in 2015, when concerns regarding denial of services were proved valid. At that time, the National Quality Forum quietly proposed a rule derived from the USPSTF recommendation that would penalize primary care physicians up to 2% of their Medicare reimbursement if they ordered screening PSAs on their patients.[13] Clearly, this would have had a chilling effect on early diagnosis of prostate cancer, and although the tsunami of objections by the urologic community thwarted this misguided initiative,[14] this clearly exemplified the need for close monitoring and immediate action to protect access to care for patients.

Although advocacy on the federal level had commenced immediately on the release of the USPSTF recommendation, the actions by the National Quality Forum and dramatic data that suggested increasing death rates from prostate cancer galvanized continued and expanded engagement.[15–18] The urologic community did not focus solely on PSA testing; historically, Congress is reluctant to act when presented with differing expert opinions, particularly when an advisory board is empowered to make policy recommendations. Instead, the urologic community aligned with other stakeholders to educate lawmakers on the process by which the USPSTF operated; remarkably, the fact that the USPSTF was able to operate without congressional oversight was surprising to legislators.

The combination of input across various specialties with engagement of patient groups proved powerful. Congressional leaders recalled the USPSTF recommendation against screening for breast cancer; in fact, based on immediate and aggressive response of breast cancer patient advocacy groups, language carving out breast cancer screening from USPSTF authority was included in the ACA. As such, there was no shortage of sympathetic members of Congress, many of whom either were prostate cancer survivors themselves or had a close relative battling the disease. Ultimately, this led to the USPSTF Transparency and Accountability Act. Rather than focusing on a single recommendation for a single disease state in a single specialty, this legislation required that the USPSTF adhere to the same transparency and oversight requirements required of every other federal advisory committee and to consider the view of content-specific experts when promulgating recommendations.

The impact of these advocacy efforts on the USPSTF process has been profound.

Although the USPSTF has engaged in its own advocacy efforts to prevent passage of the USPSTF Transparency and Accountability Act, the specter of legislative changes to their mandate has resulted in a substantial change in the process by which they promulgate recommendations, with much greater visibility into the decision-making process and inclusion of appropriate subject matter experts. The requirement to consult content experts when evaluating services. A direct consequence of these reforms was the 2018 revisitation and modification of the grade D recommendation on PSA-based prostate cancer screening to a more appropriate grade C recommendation. Efforts did not end there; in 2019, thanks to diligent advocacy efforts by urology practices within the state, New York became the first state in the United States to mandate no out-of-pocket insurance coverage for PSA testing for men over age 40.[19]

## POLITICAL ACTION COMMITTEES AND FUNDRAISING

A part of the political process that many find distasteful is fundraising; this includes both those asked for and receiving contributions. From the moment a member of Congress is sworn into office, that representative immediately must think about the next election, which in the US House of Representatives is every 2 years. A significant amount of time for all members on both sides of the aisle is devoted to fundraising efforts. And although any citizen can engage with the political process, the opportunity to interact with an elected official during a fundraising event affords the opportunity to engage in what often is a much smaller and more social forum. And although there can absolutely never be any suggestion or expectation that any political contribution can result in a legislative quid pro quo, the opportunity to present a point of view that otherwise may not be heard is invaluable.

In broad brush strokes, there are 2 general mechanisms by which fundraising is conducted, via representative entities, such as political action committees (PACs), or by direct giving. PACs are a tool under the authority of the Federal Election Commission that allow pooling of donations from a defined group of citizens so the contribution can be given in larger amounts to selected candidates. There are 2 PACs that exist in the urology community—the AUAPAC, which is associated with the AUA, and UROPAC, administered by the AACU. In general, a contributor to an organization's PAC must be a member of the organization and a US citizen. LUGPA also engages in political giving by asking for member group practices to donate to individual fundraising events to specific congressional members. By law, these 2 entities must act independently and cannot coordinate giving.

The advantage to having multiple organizations participating in the process is that it does provide multiple vehicles for political giving; this must be balanced against the possibility that political donations are split between different entities. That said, although political giving cannot be co-ordinated between organizations, messaging certainly can be. Because different urologic societies have somewhat different legislative priorities and constituencies, having similar messaging delivered from different viewpoints broadens the specialty's presence on Capitol Hill. One way to increase the volume of advocacy messages is by having it repeated by different groups throughout the year. Having a mechanism to donate gives a specialty a place at the table and a mechanism for congressional members to access opinions. AUAPAC is in its infancy but already has contributed to 24 individuals. URO-PAC has more of a history and also contributed to a similar number of lawmakers over the past year, with total contributions by its members in the 6-figures yearly. LUGPA works under a system of individual giving and not through a PAC, and its activities on the Hill have been extensive and hugely effective in favor of urology. All 3 organizations aim to distribute those contributions equally among the 2 major parties and focus on members who have been supportive of the concerns and those who are on pertinent committees of jurisdiction. These organizations advocating for urology are nonpartisan with respect to political party but are hugely partisan in favor of patients' interests and urologist members.

## THE CHANGING FACE OF PHYSICIAN ADVOCACY

One challenge facing urology is the demographic makeup of the specialty. Although it is a core focus of the urologic community to increase diversity within its ranks, historically, physicians who engage in advocacy tend to be older—for urology, this population is composed overwhelmingly of white men.[20–30] Messaging is more impactful when presented by professionals with varied backgrounds and practice environments. This is particularly important because much of the legislative work is done by legislative assistants, who themselves tend to be younger and from diverse backgrounds.

That said, efforts to enlist a more diverse group of physicians have been more complicated than just inviting individuals to participate. Younger doctors who are concerned about building their practices generally are focused on patient care and may not be fully engaged on the business and administrative aspects of their business. More senior physicians may not actively seek their opinions, and, when asked, the younger doctor may be more inclined to "go along to get along" than be viewed as a troublemaker within the practice—this is complicated further by the fact that the needs and goals of the younger physician may differ from the decision makers in the group. Given their work schedules and economic needs, unless the group specifically makes provisions for advocacy efforts, it may not be economically feasible for younger doctors to take time out of their schedules to engage in these processes.

Despite these challenges, the face of urologic advocacy has changed dramatically over the past decade. For example, at the 2020 AUA Advocacy Summit, 80 of the 300 attendees were students, residents, fellows, and young urologists, the largest number to date. The LUGPA Forward program continues to expand its membership, and opportunities for formal fellowships and informal apprenticeships in the advocacy realm continue to grow and be fully subscribed. Going forward, the urologic community needs to actively engage with medical students whose demographics are not well represented in the specialty to consider a career in urology.

## SUMMARY

The nation's health care agenda is robust, and there are a significant number of issues having an impact on urologists nationwide. With a divided electorate and multiple stakeholders competing for limited resources, the need for engagement never has been greater. This need will be amplified as lawmakers and regulatory agencies seek to shift payments from volume-based to value-based models and will seek input from subject matter experts to help guide these policies. Without question, the specialty of urology has laid a solid foundation in an impressively short period of time; the specialty needs to build on that foundation to ensure that their voice continues to be heard. That said, they cannot advocate effectively without the support and help of all involved in the care of urologic disease — voice, commitment, advocacy, and yes, financial commitment are vital to the future of the specialty.

## DISCLOSURE

The authors have nothing to disclose.

## REFERENCES

1. Combined Degrees and Early Acceptance Programs. Available at: https://www.aamc.org/data-reports/curriculum-reports/interactive-data/combined-degrees-and-early-acceptance-programs.
2. American Lithotripsy Soc. v. Thompson, 215 F. Supp. 2d 23 (D.D.C. 2002).
3. Al-Azzawi IS, Koraitim MM. Lower genitourinary trauma in modern warfare: the experience from civil violence in Iraq. Injury 2014;45(5):885–9.
4. Medicare Access and CHIP Reauthorization Act of 2010. Pub. L. 111-148, as amended by the Health Care and Education Reconciliation Act of 2010 (Pub. L. 111-152).
5. Moyer VAS. Preventive Services Task Force. Screening for prostate cancer: U.S. Preventive Services Task Force recommendation statement. Ann Intern Med 2012;157(2):120–34.
6. Statistics and Historical Comparisons. Available at: https://www.govtrack.us/congress/bills/statistics.
7. HHS Agencies & Offices. Available at: https://www.hhs.gov/about/agencies/hhs-agencies-and-offices/index.html.
8. Edney MT. Urotrauma - The Success of an AUA Legislative Initiative: A Legislative Primer. Urol Pract 2015;2(2):73–7.
9. Kapoor DA. A History of the United States preventive services task force: its expanding authority and need for reform. J Urol 2018;199(1):37–9.
10. Medicare Improvements for Patients and Providers Act of 2008 (Public Law 110–275, July 15, 2008, 122 Stat. 2494).
11. Patient protection and affordable care act, 42 U.S.C. § 18001 (2010).
12. Harris R, Lohr KN. Screening for prostate cancer: an update of the evidence for the U.S. Preventive Services Task Force. Ann Intern Med 2002;137(11):917–29.
13. Mathematica Policy Research. Non-Recommended PSA-Based Screening. Available at: https://talk aboutprostatecancer.files.wordpress.com/2015/11/psa-screening_framing-document_measure-specification_hqmf-header3.pdf.
14. CMS Response to Public Comments on Non-Recommended PSA-Based Screening Measure. Available at: http://www.cms.gov/Medicare/Quality-Initiatives-Patient-Assessment-Instruments/MMS/Downloads/eCQM-Development-and-Maintenance-for-Eligible-Professionals_CMS_PSA_Response_Public-Comment.pdf.
15. Bhindi B, Mamdani M, Kulkarni GS, et al. Impact of the U.S. preventive services task force recommendations against prostate specific antigen screening on prostate biopsy and cancer detection rates. J Urol 2015;193(5):1519.
16. Barocas DA, Mallin K, Graves AJ, et al. Effect of the USPSTF Grade D recommendation against screening for prostate cancer on incident prostate cancer diagnoses in the United States. J Urol 2015;194(6):1587.
17. Penson A, Fedewa SA, Ma J, et al. Prostate Cancer Incidence and PSA Testing Patterns in Relation to USPSTF Screening Recommendations. JAMA 2015;314(19):2054–61.
18. Hall MD, Schultheiss TE, Farino G, et al. Increase in higher risk prostate cancer cases following new screening recommendation by the US Preventive Services Task Force (USPSTF). J Clin Oncol 2015; 33(suppl 7). abstr: 143].
19. Ricks D. New York State health insurers now required to cover PSA blood test. Newsday 2019. Available at: https://www.newsday.com/news/health/psa-screening-new-law-1.27635679.
20. Washington SL 3rd, Baradaran N, Gaither TW, et al. Racial distribution of urology workforce in United States in comparison to general population. Transl Androl Urol 2018;7(4):526–34.
21. Shore N. The evolution of understanding the USPSTF: recommendations and controversy. 2018. Available at: https://The-Evolution-of-Understanding-the-USPSTF/. Accessed November 2020.
22. Andriole G, Crawford ED, Grubb RL, et al. Prostate cancer screening in the randomized Prostate, Lung, Colorectal, and Ovarian Cancer Screening Trial: mortality results after 13 years of follow-up. J Natl Cancer Inst 2012;104(2):125–32.
23. Schröder FH, Hugosson J, Roobol MJ, et al. Screening and prostate-cancer mortality in a randomized European study. N Engl J Med 2009; 360(13):1320–8.
24. Etzioni R, Tsodikov A, Mariotto A, et al. Quantifying the role of PSA screening in the US prostate cancer mortality decline. Cancer Causes Control 2008; 19(2):175–81.
25. Etzioni R, Gulati R, Cooperberg MR, et al. Limitations of basing screening policies on screening trials: The US Preventive Services Task Force and

Prostate Cancer Screening. Med Care 2013;51(4): 295–300.

26. Etzioni R, Gulati R, Tsodikov A, et al. The prostate cancer conundrum revisited: treatment changes and prostate cancer mortality declines. Cancer 2012;118(23):5955–63.

27. Carter HB, Albertsen PC, Barry MJ, et al. Early detection of prostate cancer: AUA guideline. J Urol 2013;190(2):419–26.

28. Olsson C, Anderson A, Kapoor D. Mp39-04 Initial Prostate Cancer Detection before and after United States preventive services task force recommendation on prostate cancer screening. J Urol 2016; 195(4S):e542.

29. Blair BM, Robyak H, Clark JY, et al. Impact of United States Preventive Services Task Force recommendations on prostate biopsy characteristics and disease presentation at a tertiary-care medical center. Prostate Int 2018;6(3):110–4.

30. Catalona WJ. Prostate Cancer Screening. Med Clin North Am 2018;102(2):199–214.

# Current and Future Status of Merit-Based Incentive Payment Systems

Kathleen L. Latino, MD, FACS[a],*, Deepak A. Kapoor, MD[b]

## KEYWORDS

- MIPS • MACRA • Quality payment program

## KEY POINTS

- The Quality Payment Program established by Medicare Access and CHIP Reauthorization Act (MACRA) legislation establishes the guidelines for payments now and in the future to Medicare providers.
- The program consists of 2 current pathways (Alternative Payment Models and Merit-based Incentive Payment Systems [MIPSs]) and 1 proposed future pathway (MIPS value pathways).
- The program is complex and reporting is burdensome, and both Centers for Medicare and Medicaid Services and providers are looking for ways to achieve the goals of MACRA without creating more administrative burdens.

## INTRODUCTION

The Medicare Access and CHIP Reauthorization Act (MACRA) created the Quality Payment Program (QPP), which is responsible for paying Medicare providers. The goal was to emphasize a balance between quality and cost and to assess the overall value of care delivered to the beneficiaries. Now that the QPP is in its fourth year, providers, beneficiaries, and Centers for Medicare and Medicaid Services (CMS) are reviewing its effects both for its burdens and its effects on care. The program is evolving; however, certain parts of the legislation will become absolute law in the next few years. This article is an examination of this evolution and a discussion of the future of MACRA, Alternative Payment Models (APMs), and Merit-based Incentive Payment Systems (MIPSs).

## HISTORY

The history of the current physician fee schedule began in 1992 when the resource-based relative value scale (RBRVS) was put into place by the Omnibus Budget Reconciliation Act of 1989.[1] A formula would determine what each procedure performed by physicians was worth based on different costs involved in providing the service. These costs included physician work, practice expense, and malpractice. CMS is responsible for the final fee schedule but the RUC (Relative Value Scale Update Committee) advises CMS. This committee is composed of 31 volunteer physicians whose purpose is to advise Medicare on the value of the work of a physician depending on the procedure. Specialty societies advise the RUC about proposed updates to the RBRVS. The RUC then makes the recommendations to CMS, which then addresses these revisions in its final rule every year.

The Balanced Budget Act (BBA) of 1997 included key Medicare provisions meant to assure the solvency of Medicare over an extended period of time. This assurance was to be achieved by reducing spending by limiting the growth of payments to hospitals and physicians as well as

[a] Solaris Health Holdings, LLC, 340 Broadhollow Road, Farmingdale, NY 11735, USA; [b] The Icahn School of Medicine at Mount Sinai, New York, NY, USA
* Corresponding author.
E-mail address: klatino@imppllc.com
Twitter: @Kllnd82md (K.L.L.)

Urol Clin N Am 48 (2021) 259–268
https://doi.org/10.1016/j.ucl.2021.01.004

restructuring the payment methods to rehabilitation facilities, skilled nursing facilities, home health agencies, and outpatient service agencies in the hope of improving efficiencies. Medicare managed care plans also saw a significant reduction in payments. There were also provisions to increase beneficiary premiums.[2]

One key provision of the BBA was that physicians' fee schedule was to be determined by a formula called the sustainable growth rate (SGR) payment formula. It was hoped that this formula would help to limit Medicare spending. Under the formula, if a weighted combination of annual and cumulative expenditures was less than the weighted annual and cumulative spending target for the period, the annual update was increased according to an established calculation. However, if the weighted combination of annual and cumulative spending exceeded the weighted annual cumulative spending target over a certain period, future updates were reduced to bring spending back in line with the target.[3]

For about 4 years, the expenditures were in line with the targets and the updates to the fee schedule were close to what was expected. However, eventually, starting in 2002, the expenditures were higher than the targets. Doctors were to have a 4.8% cut in 2002 and the first so-called doc fix was implemented, which temporarily delayed the cuts.[4] Congress then began to override what would have been mandated reductions with several different laws that only provided short-term relief. Most of the time these bills kept the level of payment at the current rate (0% increase) or gave a slight increase (never >2.2%). During the years leading up to 2014, there were several bills introduced in both houses that attempted to put in place a permanent fix to the SGR formula. The country faced a fiscal cliff in 2013 when the Bush tax cuts were set to expire and a set of spending cuts were going to go into effect. It was feared that the combination would throw the economy back into a recession. The spending cuts included a possible 27% cut in Medicare fees. In a last-minute deal, Congress passed the American Tax Relief Act of 2012, which kept most of the Bush tax cuts and readded the previous 39.6% tax rate for higher income earners and also included among other provisions another 1-year doc fix that avoided the 27% cut. This fix of the situation was again only temporary.[5]

In addition, in 2015 the bipartisan legislation MACRA was passed. It created the QPP, which:

- Repealed the SGR formula
- Changed the way that Medicare rewards clinicians for value rather than volume

- Streamlined the multiple quality programs under the new MIPSs
- Gave bonus payments for participation in eligible APMs

This legislation went into effect in 2017.[6]

## THE QUALITY PAYMENT PROGRAM

By statute, MACRA required CMS to begin rewarding quality, value, and outcomes and penalizing providers that do not provide such value. The QPP at its start had 2 paths for providers. Providers could either participate in an APM or participate in an MIPS. A third option is being explored by CMS for implementation within the next 2 to 5 years, called the MIPS Value Pathways. The years from 2017 to 2021 were considered transition years in the original law, and CMS was given flexibility in those years to adjust thresholds and category weights for APM participation and MIPSs. In the year 2022, by law, this flexibility will no longer be available to CMS.

### Alternative Payment Models

An APM is a method of payment based on quality and value. The purpose of an APM is to provide high-quality care in a way that is cost-efficient. There are several options under the APM model. These options include Advanced APMs, MIPS APMs, and all-payer APMs.[7]

### Advanced Alternative Payment Models

The following are necessary for an APM to qualify for status as an Advanced APM:

- Participants must use certified electronic health record (EHR) technology
- Payment for covered professional services must be based on quality measures comparable with those used in the MIPS quality performance category
- Either (1) APM is a Medical Home Model expanded under CMS Innovation Center authority, or (2) participants bear a significant financial risk
- Starting in 2020 the Advanced APM must also satisfy the 1 of the following:
  - Receive at least 50% of its Medicare Part B payments through the Advanced APM (expected to increase to 75% in year 2021)
  - See at least 35% of its Medicare patients through the Advanced APM (expected to increase to 50% in year 2021)

A qualified provider (QP) who successfully participates in an Advanced APM:

- Is exempt from MIPSs

- Qualifies for a 5% bonus based on Part B Revenues (currently this is scheduled to expire after the 2024 payment year)
- Will receive a 0.75% Part B schedule increase in 2026 (compared with 0.25% by non-APM participants)

There is the ability for an APM to achieve partial status if the entity only meets the following thresholds:

- Receives only 40% (rather than 50%) of its Medicare Part B payments through the APM
- Sees at least 25% (rather than 35%) of its Medicare Part B patients through the APM

Participants in Partial APMs can opt to participate in MIPS (but will be scored differently because of their participation in the APM). They will not receive the 5% APM bonus but may be eligible for extra MIPS APM credit.

CMS determines whether a participant meets the thresholds for participation by looking at snapshots throughout the year using Medicare administrative claims data. These data determine whether a provider is eligible as a full QP or partial QP or whether the provider is participating in an MIPS APM.

### Merit-Based Incentive Payment System Alternative Payment Models

Some clinicians do not meet the criteria for being a QP for an Advanced APM but are still participating providers during the period that is being evaluated. These clinicians have to report as MIPS providers but are scored with the APM standard. There were 10 APMs that were expected to be eligible to be MIPS APMs in 2020.

The scoring for MIPS for those subject to the APM standard eliminates the cost component because these participants are assessed for cost within the APM itself. The following is the APM standard for MIPS scoring in 2020:

- Quality: 50%
- Improvement Activities : 20%
- Promoting Interoperability : 30%
- Cost: 0%

In the proposed 2021 rule, CMS plans to replace the APM scoring standard with a new MIPS APM Performance Pathway; however, it still uses the same category weighting. It includes a 6-measure Core Quality set, the standard Promoting Interoperability measures, automatic full credit for improvement activities, and no cost measures. Those practitioners included in the APM Performance Pathway include those in MIPSs APMs

and those ACOs in the Medicare Shared Savings program.

### All-Payer Alternative Payment Models

Since 2019, clinicians can become qualified participants through an all-payer option. The qualified participants must participate in a combination of Advanced APM with Medicare and an Other-Payer APM with similar criteria to the Medicare APM.

### The Alternative Payment Model Outlook for Urology

According to CMS in performance year 2019, 195,564 clinicians were able to reach status as Qualified APM Participants in an Advanced APM and 27,995 clinicians received partial status. This number was an increase from 183,306 in 2018 for full status in Advanced APMs and 47 with partial status in 2018.

In 2017, less than 1% of urologists were participants in an Advanced APM. With that in mind, Large Urology Group Practice Association (LUGPA) presented a proposed APM centered on active surveillance for men with newly diagnosed prostate cancer. In accordance with MACRA, in December 2017 the proposal was presented to the PTAC (Payment Model Technical Advisory Committee). PTAC did not recommend testing of the APM to HHS (Health and Human Services) Secretary Azar.[8] LUGPA has continued to engage with the Secretary in order to move toward modification of the process of APM adoption. At this time, only 1 surgical specialty APM model is in place (Comprehensive Care for Joint Replacement Model).

## MERIT-BASED INCENTIVE PAYMENT SYSTEMS

For those who were not eligible to participate in an Advanced APM, the other path in the QPP is an MIPS.

Each year CMS establishes a minimum participation threshold for clinicians for MIPS based on Medicare Part B billing and the number of patients seen. **Table 1** shows the thresholds through 2020.

In addition, beginning in 2019, to be eligible clinicians must deliver at least 200 covered professional services.[9]

Clinicians may participate either as an individual or as a group. A group is a set of clinicians who share a common TIN (Tax Identification Number). Beginning in 2018, CMS allowed the option of individual clinicians to form and participate in MIPS as a virtual group. The virtual group is only applicable to clinicians in groups that have 10 or fewer eligible

| Table 1 | | |
|---|---|---|
| Minimal participation thresholds for merit-based incentive payment systems | | |
| Year | Medicare Spend Threshold ($) | Part B Patient Threshold |
| 2017 | 30,000 | 100 patients |
| 2018–2020 | 90,000 | 200 patients |

clinicians. The virtual group establishes its own TIN for MIPS reporting, which allows small groups to pool resources for reporting and aggregate data for reporting on quality measures. There must be a written agreement among the participants in a virtual group that includes all the rules established by CMS for forming a virtual group.

The MIPS program includes 4 distinct categories. These categories are Quality, Advancing Care Information (formally Meaningful Use and now titled Promoting Interoperability), Improvement Activities, and Cost. These 4 categories contribute to a final score. The weight of each category changes yearly. The purpose of the changes is to promote balancing quality and cost as the program progresses by increasing the contribution of the Cost category and decreasing the contribution of the Quality category. By law, the Cost and Quality performance categories must be equally weighed at 30% beginning in the 2022 performance year.[10]

### Quality

The assessment of the quality of care is based on certain measures of performance. These measures are created by CMS as well as other stakeholders, such as specialty groups. Newer measures have been developed by specialty societies so that specialty clinicians have measures that are more relevant to their practices. It takes several years to develop historical benchmarks, and therefore these measures contribute minimal points for the clinician in the first 2 to 3 years they are available.

The following are the key points to achieving success in the Quality category:

- Each clinician, group, or virtual group must report on at least 6 quality measures.
- One of the measures must be an outcome or high-priority measure.
- The reporting period is 365 days.
- There is a threshold for completeness of data established yearly by CMS.
  - The provider or group must submit data on a certain percentage of eligible patients or encounters for each measure. For 2018, this was 60%, and 70% for 2020.
- The eligible encounters or patients that meet the measure represent the denominator for the score, and the numerator is the number of patients or encounters that fulfill the criteria of the measure.
- CMS provides benchmarks for each measure based on historical data it has received. These benchmarks provide the basis for the score received for each measure (0–10). Measures that do not have enough historical data and therefore do not have benchmarks have a maximum score of 3. In 2021, CMS proposed not to use historical benchmarks because it is thought the data for 2020 will not be accurate because of the pandemic. Instead, performance-based benchmarks will be used, meaning the benchmarks will be based on combined actual data submitted for the year 2020 and 2021.
- Some measures are considered topped out, which occurs when there is little room for improvement for performance from previous years. Some of the topped-out measures have a maximum score of 7, whereas others require 100% to achieve a top score of 10, with anything less than that receiving a score of 6 or less. In 2020, 61 measures were designated as topped out.
- One bonus point is available for each high-priority measure reported after the first one reported.
- One bonus point is available for each measure reported via certified EHR technology (CEHRT) 2015 EMR using end-to-end reporting.
- The maximum number of points for quality is 60.[11]

There are very few urology-specific measures. Most of the measures that are used by urology practices have either been developed for primary care or general surgery. The American Urological Association (AUA) is promoting urology-specific measures through the AQUA (AUA Quality) Registry. However, only 2 urology-specific measures were available on the CMS measures list. These measures are combination androgen deprivation therapy in patients with high-risk prostate cancer receiving radiation (AUA measure), which is topped out in 2020, and IPSS or AUA-SI change 6 to 12 months after diagnosis of benign prostatic hyperplasia (LUGPA and the Oregon Institute), which has no benchmarks and therefore has a maximum point score of 3. These measures leave providers looking for other appropriate measures in other specialty sets, such as general surgery, gynecology, and oncology.

## Promoting Interoperability

This category replaced Meaningful Use, which was part of the Health Information Technology for Economic and Clinical Health (HITECH) Act. HITECH proposed meaningful use of interoperable EHRs throughout the United States health care delivery system as a critical national goal.[12] The measures for Promoting Interoperability have been based on the CEHRT of the EHR used by clinician or group. For 2017 and 2018, many EHRs had not been certified for 2015, so a set of transition objectives and measures were available for such clinicians. If the EHR used by the clinicians was CEHRT 2015, then a different set of measures were applied. Beginning in the year 2019, CEHRT 2015 was required for participation in the Promoting Interoperability category.

There are many exceptions for this category, including clinician types such as advanced practice practitioners, allied professionals (physical, occupational, and speech-language therapists; clinical psychologists; and registered dieticians). Also included are ASC and hospital-based clinicians and non–patient-facing clinicians.

In addition, practices of clinicians may request an exception if:

- The practice is small
- The EHR in use is decertified
- There are Internet connectivity issues
- There are extreme and uncontrollable circumstances, such as a disaster, practice closure, or severe financial distress
- The practice has no control over the availability of CEHRT

The practice or clinician must submit a hardship exception by December 31 of the performance year.

The reporting period for Promoting Interoperability is any continuous 90-day performance period. The following are the measures for performance year 2020.

1. E-prescribing (worth up to 10 points)
2. Query of prescription drug monitoring program (bonus measure, worth 5 points)
3. Support electronic referral loops by sending health information (worth up to 20 points)
4. Support electronic referral loops by receiving and incorporating health information (worth up to 20 points)
5. Provide patients electronic access to their health information (worth up to 40 points)
6. Report to 2 different public health agencies or clinical data registries (worth 10 points)

There are exceptions to all of these measures (except for providing electronic access) based on volume of patients or availability of registries or agencies. If the EHR of a practice cannot support some of the measures, the points sometimes can be reassigned to other measures.

In addition to the measures listed earlier, the clinician or practice must:

- Use CEHRT 2015 functionality (certified by the last day of the performance period)
- Submit "Yes" to the prevention of information blocking attestations
- Submit "Yes" to ONC direct review attestation
- Submit "Yes" to performance of a security risk analysis in the performance year

The scoring for Promoting Interoperability is as follows.

Measures 1, 3, 4, and 5 listed earlier are scored based a numerator and denominator. The scoring is then based on the percentage achieved for the measure. Registries can usually provide an estimated score but the scores are based on the percentage, but the final score is based on how the clinician or group performs against others submitting data. The other measures are simple attestations.

The maximum score for Promoting Interoperability is 100 points.

Promoting Interoperability accounts for 25% of the final MIPS score.[13]

## Improvement Activities

Improvement Activities are meant to show participation in activities that improve clinical practice.

The Improvement Activities are divided into those that are high weighted and those that are medium weighted. In order to receive the maximum points for this category, the clinician or group must attest to either:

- Two high-weighted activities
- One high-weighted and 2 medium-weighted activities, or
- Four medium-weighted activities

For group reporting, 50% of the clinicians must participate in the activity. The reporting period for this category is a continuous 90-day period. For 2020, there are a total of 104 Improvement Activities across the following categories:

- Expanded Practice Access
- Population Management
- Care Coordination
- Beneficiary Engagement
- Patient Safety and Practice Assessment
- Achieving Health Equity
- Behavioral and Mental Health

Improvement Activities are worth 15% of the total MIPS score in 2020. With the variety of activities available, most clinicians and groups can easily achieve a maximum score in this category.

## Cost

There are no submission data by clinicians or groups for the Cost category.

The calculation of cost is based on formulas under 3 different Cost performance category measures. These include Total cost per capita cost, Medicare spending per beneficiary clinician, and episode-based attribution. The calculations of cost are based on formulas that in the past did not always distinguish the clinician who was responsible for most of the care of the patient. These calculations have now been changed. For instance, the total per-capita cost now excludes nonprimary care services (eg, surgical) and certain specialty services. It also attributes costs to the TIN responsible for most of the events for the patient.

Episode attribution is either medical or surgical. For a medical episode, the episode is attributed to the TIN billing at least 30% of the inpatient Evaluation and Management (EM) services on Part B claims during the inpatient stay and is attributed to each clinician within the TIN that bills at least 1 EM service during the episode. For a surgical episode, the episode is attributed to the clinician who performed the procedure and the TIN of the that clinician.

Cost accounted for 0% of the final score in the initial MIPS year. The percentage that cost has contributed to the final MIPS score has slowly increased and for 2020 is up to 15%. By law, this must be at 30% by 2022.[14] Most providers have difficulty understanding the cost formulas and, more importantly find that there is little that can be done to affect the final score in this category.

## Submission of Data and Final Merit-Based Incentive Payment System Score

Data may be submitted for the QPP in several ways:

- Qualified Clinical Data Registry
- MIPS Clinical Quality Measures (CQMs)
- Electronic CQMs: requires use of data from an EHR that is CEHRT 2015
- Medicare Part B claims (for small practices <16 clinicians)
- CMS Web interface (CMS plans to sunset this in 2021 under the proposed rule)
- CAHPS for MIPS survey, which is an optional measure that entities can use to evaluate the patient experience

Before 2019, individuals could only submit data via 1 method. However, in 2019, CMS allowed more flexibility in that data could be submitted via multiple methods and be aggregated for the final MIPS score.

The final MIPS score for a clinician or group is based on a composite score for the 4 categories. Groups or clinicians can apply for a redistribution between categories for hardships. For instance, this application can occur for the Promoting Interoperability category when a practice has Internet problems, or the EHR does not maintain its certification. Also, if a practice is involved in a natural disaster, it can file for hardship relief. For 2020, because of coronavirus disease 2019 (COVID-19), practices can apply for reweighting of any of the categories to 0%. CMS provides guidance each year on allowable hardship cases.[15] Each year the performance threshold increases. The performance threshold is the minimum number of points that must be achieved (out of a possible 100) to prevent receiving a negative adjustment in the payment year (**Table 2**).

For example, in 2021, the clinician's or group's MIPS score must be 50 or more to avoid a penalty. To give an example of the scoring for 2021:

Quality maximum points toward MIPS is 40. A score of 54 out of the allowable 60 points for MIPS results in a Quality score of 36 ($0.90 \times 40$) toward the MIPS score. Scoring 90 out of 100 points for Promoting Interoperability results in a score of 22.5 ($0.9 \times 25$) points toward the final MIPS score for Promoting Interoperability. A score for improvement activities of 40 out of 40 results in 15 points toward the final MIPS score.

The score before including Cost would then be 73.5. CMS then would assign a score out of 20 for the Cost component. The final MIPS score in this example would be maximum of 93.5.

The MIPS score is then used to calculate payment adjustments for the year 2 years after the performance year. The MIPS score for 2021 will affect payments for the year 2023.

MIPS payments adjustments must be revenue neutral, meaning that the total negative adjustment

**Table 2**
**Performance thresholds and category scoring percentages**

| Year | Performance Threshold | Quality (%) | Promoting Interoperability (%) | Improvement Activities (%) | Cost (%) |
|------|----------------------|-------------|-------------------------------|----------------------------|----------|
| 2017 | 3 | 60 | 25 | 15 | 0 |
| 2018 | 15 | 50 | 25 | 15 | 10 |
| 2019 | 30 | 45 | 25 | 15 | 15 |
| 2020 | 45 | 45 | 25 | 15 | 15 |
| 2021(proposed) | 50 | 40 | 25 | 15 | 20 |
| 2022(by law) | 70 | 30 | 25 | 15 | 30 |

must equal the total positive adjustment. **Table 3** shows the maximum possible adjustments as well as the real adjustments for the first 3 years of MIPS.

To understand why the maximum positive adjustments predicted by MACRA are not what is actually requires an understand of how the payment adjustments are determined. **Table 4** shows the participation numbers for 2018 and 2019 (excluding those participating in MIPS APM).[16]

Most negative MIPS payments to date have resulted from individually eligible clinicians who do not submit data. There are instances of CMS applying the Extreme and Uncontrollable Circumstances exception when clinicians are located in a CMS-designated region affected by an uncontrollable event (such as a natural disaster). These clinicians receive a neutral payment adjustment.

MIPS-eligible clinicians with a score of 30.01 to 74.99 in performance year 2019 are also receiving 0% payment adjustment in 2021. MIPS-eligible clinicians with a final score more than 75.00 are eligible for an additional positive adjustment. Although the exception performance group is not subject to budget neutrality, there are only certain funds available to distribute to this group. Therefore, the positive adjustment for 2021 in this group ranges from 0.09% to 1.79%, which is far less than the expected adjustment when MACRA was first introduced.

## THE FUTURE OF ALTERNATIVE PAYMENT MODELS AND MERIT-BASED INCENTIVE PAYMENT SYSTEMS

Both CMS and clinicians have used the transition period to assess MACRA. At the time of its passing, Congress's goal was to improve the quality of care and at the same time provide this quality care with value. That balance between quality and cost is what drives the QPP.

From the outset, MIPSs have been a clerical burden for providers who participate in the QPP via this option. Performance in the Quality measures is often related to the ability to document in the EHR rather the true quality of care for patients. Practitioners do not really have control over the cost of care of patients yet the formula. Until the current proposed formula, there were costs attributed to providers even in instances when the provider had no control over certain costs. The current methods do not seem to be driving quality and controlling costs as expected.

Both CMS and stakeholders have recognized that adjustments need to be made to the program as it now exists. The Final Rule for 2021 addresses some of these concerns. In the 2021 Final Rule, CMS expands on its goals after the transition period for the QPP. One key point that is stated

**Table 3**
**Adjustments and incentives for quality payment program by year**

| Performance Year | Payment Year | Maximum Negative/Positive Adjustment (%) | Predicted Maximum Incentive (%) | Actual Maximum Incentive (%) |
|------------------|--------------|------------------------------------------|----------------------------------|------------------------------|
| 2017 | 2019 | −4/+4 | 2.3 | 1.88 |
| 2018 | 2020 | −5/+5 | 2.05 | 1.68 |
| 2019 | 2021 | −7/+7 | 4.69 | 1.79 |
| 2020 | 2022 | −9/+9 | TBA | TBA |
| 2021 | 2023 | −9/+9 | TBA | TBA |

**Table 4**
**Merit-based incentive payment system participation numbers outside of merit-based incentive payment system alternative payment models**

|  | 2018 | 2019 |
|---|---|---|
| Total clinicians receiving an MIPS score and payment adjustment (negative, positive, or neutral) | 559,230 | 538,186 |
| Clinicians with final score above exception threshold (%) | 73.83 | 74.00 |
| Clinicians above the performance threshold and below the exceptional threshold (%) | 22.10 | 20.02 |
| Clinicians with a final score at the performance threshold (%) | 0.74 | 5.43 |
| Clinicians with a final score below the performance threshold (%) | 3.30 | 0.55 |

numerous times is that the QPP is intended to pay for health care services in a way that drives value by linking performance on cost, quality, and the patient's experience of care.

In the Final Rule of 2020, CMS had intended to initiate MIPS Value Pathways (MVPs) in 2021. The definition of an MVP in the rule is a subset of measures and activities established through rule making.[17] The year 2021 was intended to be a transition year for MVPs; however, because of the COVID-19 pandemic, the proposal for initial MVPs will be delayed until at least the 2022 performance year. MVPs are expected to be a bridge to participation in Advanced APMs. CMS has used the 2021 rule to expand on its plan to develop MVPs. It addresses comments of stakeholders and has given detail as to what will be key provisions in the development of the MVPs. The provisions are guided by a set of principles:

- Using measures that have meaning to clinicians and connecting measures between the 4 MIPS categories with the hope of limiting clinicians' burden
- The measures and activities must result in providing comparative performance data that are valuable to patients and caregivers (including the development of subgroup reporting)
- Include measures selected using the Meaningful Measures approach, and include patient voices in the development when possible

- Include measures from APMs in an effort to reduce barriers to APM participation
- Support the transition to digital quality measures: digital quality measures would be measures that would be reported directly from the EHRs, health information exchange, registries, and similar entities

In addition to value and cost, the rule emphasizes the role of the patient experience in the development of MVPs. One of the issues addressed with MVPs is to allow different subgroups of physicians to report separately, which will allow patients to evaluate physicians in multi-specialty groups by the individual specialty of the physician. In the current system, when any group reports as a group in MIPS, the final score is attributable to each member. Patients are unable to evaluate an individual physician using the MIPS metrics. By having subgroups report separately in the MVPs, it is thought that CMS is attempting to move away from group reporting to individual reporting for certain metrics so that patients can evaluate an individual provider.

CMS is requesting stakeholders, in particular specialty societies and experts, to begin the development of MVPs and has specified in the 2021 rule the intent of MVPs and the key points that must be included in the structure of an MVP. The most important points that are addressed in the rule are the link between quality and cost and the ability of MVPs to serve as a link to the participation of providers in Advanced APMs. CMS also has heard from providers about the burden of MIPS reporting. An example of the burden for urologists is that there are only 2 quality measures that are specific for urology, neither of which had benchmarks to allow optimal scoring. Urologists must then align themselves with measures that do not really address the quality of care in a urologic practice. CMS believes that, by allowing specialty societies to contribute to the development of MVPs, this will allow specialists to participate in a pathway that addresses cost and quality similar to an Advanced APM.

One of the other provisions of interest is the inclusion of patients in the development of MVPs. CMS believes that patients should have a voice in the process and is proposing that stakeholders use various processes to include the patient voice, including satisfaction surveys, focus groups, listening sessions, and patient interviews. The proposal includes the patient voice as a prerequisite for the development of MVPs.

The MVP process will be complex and, recognizing this, CMS proposes that a template will be provided to assist in the development of MVPs. By using a template, MVP developers will be assured that benchmarks are met during the development process. For example, there may be new quality measures introduced with a particular MVP that has not been previously used. The developer will use the template to ensure that the measure meets the criteria that makes the measure meaningful and relevant both from a data analytical standpoint and a reporting standpoint.[18]

As MACRA moves forward, it seems that participation in Advanced APMs will be difficult for most urologists. MVPs provide an opportunity for urologists to engage in the process of development of measures that are relevant to urologic practice rather than trying to squeeze urologic practice into measures and pathways better suited for other specialties or primary care. It is important that these societies and stakeholders are engaged early in this process so that measurement of urologic care and its value is about urologists and their patients. Because the cost of care is obviously an important component of MVPs and MIPS going forward, urologists will have to embrace concepts and ideas that include this in any pathway or model in which there is participation. The first 5 years of MIPS was meant to be a transition and the sixth year is approaching, and at that time quality and cost will have equal footing and all providers will need to embrace that concept going forward.

## CLINICS CARE POINT

- As urologic practices transition to value-based care models, it is important that the use of MVPs will not only allow urologic physicians to report on MIPS measures in a more streamlined manner but will also include the patient voice in their care, which is a key component to the pathways.

## DISCLOSURE

The authors have no relationship with a commercial company that has a direct financial interest in this subject matter, and have nothing to disclose.

## REFERENCES

1. Omnibus Budget Reconciliation Act of 1989: Report of the Committee on the Budget, House of Representatives to Accompany H.R. 3299, a Bill to Provide for Reconciliation Pursuant to Section 5 of the Concurrent Resolution on the Budget for the Fiscal Year 1990 Together with Supplemental and Additional Views. 1989.

2. Hahn J, Blom K. The Medicare access and CHIP Reauthorization Act of 2015. Congressional Research Service; 2015.

3. Hahn J. The sustainable growth rate(SGR) and Medicare physician payments: Frequently Asked Questions. Congressional Research Service; 2014.

4. Swanson, Adam. Medicare Sustainable Growth Rate Formula and Doc Fix Explained. Available at: https://www.thenationalcouncil.org/. Accessed October 25, 2020.

5. Levit M, Crandall-Hollick M, Hahn J, et al. The "fiscal cliff" and the American Taxpayer Relief Act of 2012. Congressional Research Service R42884; 2013.

6. Medicare Access and CHIP Reauthorization Act, HR 2-2, 114th Congress (2015). Available at: https://www.congress.gov/bill/114th-congress/house2-2. Accessed October 21, 2020.

7. Qpp.cms.gov. APMs overview. Available at: https://qpp.cms.gov/apms/overview. Accessed October 22, 2020.

8. Kapoor D, Shore N, Kirsch G, et al. The LUGPA alternative payment model for initial therapy of newly diagnosed patients with organ-confined prostate cancer: rationale and development. Rev Urol 2017; 19(4):235–45.

9. qpp.cms.gov How MIPs Eligibility is Determined. Available at: https://qpp.cms.gov/mips/how-eligibility-is-determined. Accessed October 25, 2020.

10. qpp.cms.gov 2021 QPP Proposed Rule Fact Sheet. Accessed October 25, 2020.

11. MIPS Quality Quick Start Guide. 2020. Available at: qpp.com.gov. Accessed October 26, 2020.

12. cdc.gov. Public Health and Promoting Interoperability Programs. Available at: https://www.cdc.gov/ehrmeaningfuluse/introduction.html. Accessed October 25, 2020.

13. qpp.cms.gov. Promoting Interoperability Requirement: Traditional MIPS Requirements. Available at: https://qpp.cms.gov/mips/promoting-interoperability. Accessed October 26, 2020.

14. qpp.com.gov MIPS 2020 Cost Performance Category Quick Start Guide. Available at: https://qpp.cms.gov/mips/cost. Accessed October 27, 2020.

15. qpp.com.gov 2020 Quality Payment Program Exceptions Application Fact Sheet. Accessed October 27, 2020.

16. CMS. Quality Payment Program Participation in 2019: Results At-a-Glance. Accessed October 31, 2020.

17. Department of Health and Human Services and Centers for Medicare and Medicaid Services. Medicare program; CY2020 revisions to payment Policies under the physician Fee schedule and other changes to Part B payment Policies Medicare shared Savings program Requirements; Medicaid promoting Interoperability program Requirements for eligible professionals; Establishment of an Ambulance data Collection system; updates to the quality payment program; Medicare Enrollment of the Opioid Treatment programs and Enhancements to provider Enrollment

Regulations Concerning Self-Referral law advisory opinion Regulations final rule; and Coding and payment for evaluation and Management, Observation and provision of Self-Administered Esketamine; final and Interim rules. Washington, DC: Federal Register Online via the Government Publishing office; 2019. Accessed November 2, 2020.

18. Revisions to Payment Policies under the Medicare Physician Fee Schedule, Quality Payment Program and Other Revisions to Part B for CY 2021. Proposed Rule. Available at: https://www.cms.gov/medicaremedicare-fee-service-paymentphysicianfeeschedpfs-federal-regulation-notices/cms-1734-p. Accessed October 31, 2020.

# Finance 101 for Physicians

Christopher G. Stappas, J.D, CFP®

## KEYWORDS

- Financial planning for physicians • Retirement planning for physicians • Finance 101 for physicians
- Insurance planning • Estate planning • Tax-reduction strategies • Legacy planning
- Wealth preservation

## KEY POINTS

- Although physicians enjoy extensive educational backgrounds, financial planning typically is not a significant component of the curricula they have completed.
- Many physicians could benefit from greater financial acumen, and their preparation for retirement might be lacking in light of their relatively high-income levels.
- Three pillars of financial planning for physicians include (1) protecting themselves, their families, and their assets; (2) reducing their taxes; and (3) growing their wealth.
- The capstone to these 3 pillars is creating a holistic financial plan, whether it is designed by a financial professional or is personally crafted based on a comprehensive evaluation of financial health.
- The lost benefits of compound growth, tax deferral, and tax reduction never can be replaced, so creating a financial plan early and reviewing it often exponentially increase the odds of success.

As "Finance 101" implies, this article is meant to provide physicians with the basic building blocks to understand and manage their finances. Although physicians enjoy extensive educational backgrounds overall, financial planning typically is not a significant component of the curricula they complete. A 2017 study published by the *International Journal of Medical Education* revealed a mean quiz score of just 52% among 422 residents and fellows, who answered 20 questions on personal finance and 28 questions about their own financial planning, attitudes, and debt.[1]

This study concluded, "Residents and fellows had low financial literacy and investment risk tolerance, high debt, and deficits in their financial preparedness. Adding personal financial education to the medical education curriculum would benefit trainees. Providing education in areas such as budgeting, estate planning, investment strategies, and retirement planning early in training can offer significant long-term benefits."

Clearly, a need exists for greater financial awareness and knowledge among physicians.

But, in some ways, effectively navigating financial life can be similar to how physicians work with patients. If a patient asks for advice on how to optimize his or her health, initially, some small but impactful suggestions are given in the hope that the person would implement 1 or 2 and see a positive impact.

This advice could include identifying basic pillars of health, such as maintaining a healthy diet, avoiding smoking, exercising regularly, and receiving annual physical examinations. In the same vein, this article identifies basic pillars of a sound financial strategy, in the hope of providing some actionable items that may offer immediate practical benefits.

These pillars are based on my extensive experience working with physician clients over the past 29 years. Regardless of their specialty, many physicians tend to have similar primary goals that can be categorized into 3 broad areas: (1) protecting themselves, their families, and their assets; (2) reducing their taxes; and (3) growing their wealth. This article addresses these considerations, while

Summit Financial, LLC, 4 Campus Drive, Parsippany, NJ 07054, USA
*E-mail address:* cstappas@sfr1.com

Urol Clin N Am 48 (2021) 269–277
https://doi.org/10.1016/j.ucl.2020.12.005
0094-0143/21/© 2020 Elsevier Inc. All rights reserved.

also providing suggestions on how best to achieve these goals and tips on how to avoid common mistakes.

## PILLAR 1: PROTECTING FAMILY, PERSON, AND ASSETS

Financial planning starts with identifying assets and creating a plan that protects them. Quite simply, a physician is his or her most important asset, and a comprehensive plan is needed to properly protect a professional's future.

### Protecting Family

For high earners like physicians, their ability to earn a consistent and reliable income often is their family's greatest asset. Losing that asset—due to either death or disability—could be devastating to their family's financial health. Fortunately, there are several key measures physicians can take to assure they, and their families, are well protected.

The most basic actionable item is to ensure that the proper planning documents are in place. These include a will, which enables beneficiary access to assets and specifies child guardianship. Additionally, a power of attorney of property allows a spouse or another representative to handle financial affairs in the event of incapacity. A health care directive enables an authorized representative to make medical decisions in the event of incapacity, with a living will dictating end-of-life wishes if that incapacitation is associated with no hope of recovery. Any competent estate planning attorney can draft these 4 documents, which commonly are done as a package for the entire family, easily and cost-effectively.

Throughout my career, I have come across numerous successful and wealthy individuals who did not have a will despite having families. This is rectified easily: simply find an attorney, make the call, and get it done. Whenever meeting someone without a will, I tend to paint a vivid picture of the nightmare scenario that would unfold for the spouse and children if the individual dies unexpectedly—because the spouse would need to go through the court system to gain control of and access to their assets. This is a time consuming and expensive process that could easily be avoided, eliminating the burden on already grieving spouse and children.

It also is important to implement proper planning documents for children who have reached the age of majority, which is 18 in most states. At the very least, it is prudent for them to have health care directives. Physicians know the importance of these documents. When children go to college and potentially face medical emergencies, there could be instances where parents cannot properly access information and authorize care for them because they lack legal authorization to do so.

Additionally, verify that the beneficiaries on insurance policies, individual retirement accounts (IRAs), and pension plans are named properly (this is especially important following a divorce, birth, death, or other life-altering event). There have been cases when, after a divorce and remarriage, the husband never changed the beneficiary of his IRA from his ex-wife to his new spouse or to his biological children. As a result, the ex-wife legally was entitled to the husband's IRA after his unexpected passing, with his children and new spouse having no legal recourse.

### Protecting Self

From a life insurance standpoint, the first step is to determine an appropriate amount of coverage. This analysis should be customized based on each individual's personal situation. How much indebtedness is there? Should this debt be paid off in the event of untimely death? What is the earning ability of the spouse and the value of other family assets. How many children need to be cared for and what are their anticipated costs for education? What income is required to maintain the family's lifestyle? How much of a legacy should be left to children after spousal demise?

I take all of my clients through a comprehensive analysis to determine the amount of insurance they truly need based on the answers to these questions. At the least, it is prudent to have enough life insurance to pay off all debts (mortgages, student loans, and so forth) and still retain enough cash to fund an investment portfolio that replaces the income lost due to death. For example, a $100,000-a-year earner who enjoyed a 4% portfolio return needs a $2.5 million investment account earning a 4% return to replace that income ($2,500,000 × .04 = $100,000) and keep the investment principal in tact.

After determining an appropriate amount of coverage, identify the best insurance portfolio design based on affordability. Term life insurance is the least expensive and can be purchased for guaranteed time periods, such as 10 years, 15 years, 20 years, and 30 years. Although term insurance is relatively inexpensive, it offers no cash accumulation and disappears without value at the end of the designated time period. In a sense, obtaining term insurance is like renting an apartment rather than buying a house.

There also are permanent insurance strategies that offer coverage throughout the life of the holder. These strategies can be structured to provide additional retirement benefits and are beneficial from a tax perspective, because life insurance proceeds are 100% income tax–free to beneficiaries. When designed properly, these polices also can be utilized to generate tax-free distributions during retirement, thus creating an additional lifetime benefit.

It is wise to conduct a thorough insurance analysis with a competent and qualified advisor to determine the most appropriate insurance portfolio design. And then, make sure that the appropriate coverage is implemented. Unfortunately, I have had my share of conversations with grieving spouses who were not clients and could not understand why their partner had insufficient life insurance to meet the basic needs of their families.

The consequence of the failure of basic planning is a family faced with a lifetime of financial burden in addition to the emotional grief. For premium payments of just a few hundred dollars per month, which would have had negligible impact on the family's lifestyle, a lifetime of hardship could have been avoided. The simple fact is this: nobody ever plans to die prematurely or unexpectedly, but, unfortunately, it happens all the time. Thus, after ensuring the proper documents are in place, assessing the status of and securing appropriate life insurance coverage are the next most important steps in financial planning for professionals.

Statistically, experiencing disability is much more likely than premature death. Although a life policy typically is the first consideration when assessing insurance needs, another often overlooked key aspect to financial planning is proper disability coverage. There are 2 broad types of disability policies to consider: individual and group. Individual coverage can be obtained independently, and, although it usually is more expensive, often can provide additional benefits that stay with the policyholder, regardless of workplace. Group coverage relies on employment status or society membership, and, although it generally is less expensive, it is also less customizable because the terms and rates are negotiated for a cohort of individuals. A critical point is that this coverage is contingent on continued membership in the group; the policy may not be transferable and a physician may lose this coverage upon leaving a practice.

An important nuance for physicians to consider regarding potential disability is "own occupation" coverage. Those with highly specialized occupations should have this type of insurance because it extends specific and long-term benefits when they are unable to carry out the job they were trained to perform. For example, consider a surgeon who suffers a hand injury and no longer can fulfill his or her job responsibilities. Own-occupation coverage ensures that person still receives a disability benefit, even if he or she also chooses to receive income through lecturing or conducting research following the injury.

### Protecting Assets

Another protection to have in place is excess liability (umbrella) coverage. This typically is purchased through a homeowner's insurance policy and designed to provide coverage in the event someone is injured by a family member or at a domicile. A good rule of thumb is to have coverage similar to net worth. For most physicians, a policy of at least $3 million to $5 million would be prudent and economically feasible. Typically, the cost to increase coverage by an additional $1 million to $2 million is not that significant and probably worth it from a risk management perspective.

Additionally, proper home and auto insurance should be obtained as well as reviewed on an annual basis to assure that appropriate coverage and deductibles are included. It also can be simple to restructure these policies to provide maximum cost savings. For instance, while reviewing a client's insurance coverage, I found that the homeowner's policy included a $1000 deductible. This was much more expensive than a $5000 deductible would have been, and it is rare for a policy owner to submit a homeowner's claim for less than $5000. Simply by increasing the deductible to $5000, that client was able to enjoy a lower premium bill every year without significantly increasing risk exposure.

Many other asset-protection strategies could be sensible as well but are beyond the scope of this article. The tips provided in this article are viewed best as a helpful primer on the topic.

### Protect the Future

### Protect the business

For business owners, there are additional considerations to keep in mind. For example, owners should ensure that the practice and any owned real estate associated with it are classified within a legal entity (limited liability company [LLC], professional LLC, S corporation, partnership, and so forth) and not owned individually. This measure can help protect personal assets in case of a business liability event. It is wise to consult with an attorney to determine the most applicable legal structure.

### Start exit planning early

In a practice owned jointly with partners, it also is important to have buy–sell agreements in place, because, if 1 partner suddenly dies, a tremendous strain can be put on the practice, causing business interruptions and necessitating the hiring of a new physician.

Likewise, if the deceased was an income-producing active partner, consideration must be given to spouse and family. Any assets (including accounts receivable) and good will generated over a professional career have value, and that value should be tendered as appropriate to the deceased partner's estate. Accordingly, it is prudent to negotiate a partnership agreement that specifies the group's legal obligations under such circumstances—again, leaving this to a bereaved spouse and family adds insult to injury. Fortunately, such agreements can be funded with inexpensive term insurance on each of the partners. It makes sense to review a practice's buy–sell agreement every 3 years to 5 years to ensure it is relevant to the business scenario and partnership composition.

## PILLAR 2: TAX PLANNING

One of the most consistent messages I deliver to clients is the importance of mitigating and eliminating taxes whenever possible. Successfully achieving this objective year in and year out, throughout all aspects of finances, offers one of the best avenues to accumulating wealth.

Even the most cursory perusal of current events reveals an ever-loudening drumbeat in this country to increase the tax burden on those who produce the most. Such tax raises likely are a matter of when, not if. Given these circumstances, it is prudent to not delay tax planning, to appropriately take advantage of every opportunity to decrease tax burden as long as such vehicles exist.

### First, Maximize Retirement Contributions

The importance of maximizing annual contributions to a practice retirement plan (if one exists) cannot be overstated. In 2020, a typical 401(k)/profit-sharing plan may allow a maximum annual contribution of $57,000, or $63,500 for those over age 50.[2]

This is a key difference between income and wealth: what matters is not what is earned but what is kept. Sometimes, a client says that he or she cannot afford to contribute the maximum amount. But whatever is not contributed up to the maximum is considered ordinary income and is fully taxable. Due to the graduated tax system, that $57,000 comes off the top. A physician

earning $500,000 is in a 35% federal tax bracket; so, assuming a state tax rate of 9%, the $57,000 (earned) really is netting just $31,920 (kept).

Given these figures, the client can make a truly educated decision. Is it better to have $57,000 growing in a tax-deferred pension plan for the next 10 years or 20 years until retirement or to have $31,920 now, which comes out to $2660 net cash per month? When I conduct retirement funding analyses with clients, long-term wealth accumulation in a tax-deferred pension plan almost always emerges as a better option than forgoing the maximum deduction and investing that after-tax money in a taxable investment account—if the funds ever get invested at all rather than simply being spent.

Countless clients have told me they never seem to miss the pension money that was automatically deducted from their pay, and they never felt as though they had to compromise their lifestyle. But if that money is not contributed to the pension plan, it always seems to be spent on something else and not utilized to accumulate wealth in another investment account.

For practice owners, it is important to be aware of all available pension strategies. Numerous designs (cash balance plans, defined benefit plans, and so forth) can enable physicians to make hundreds of thousands of dollars of tax-deductible contributions each year. All these plans also require, however, that certain mandatory contributions be made for employees. So, the relative cost and benefit to the practice owner can vary greatly, depending on the number of employees and owners as well as their respective ages and salaries.

It is prudent to engage a retirement specialist to determine the different plan options available and the most appropriate design. For a physician practice, I was able to implement a 401(k)/profit-sharing/cash balance plan design that allowed a 60-year-old owner to contribute more than $290,000 annually and a 50-year-old owner to contribute more than $195,000 each year.

Contributions of this size create significant benefits for the physician owners. Not only do substantial allocations continue to grow tax-deferred for decades, but the large tax deductions can also move the physicians into lower tax brackets and reduce their current income tax liability.

### Next, Minimize or Eliminate the Tax Burden on Personal, Nonpension Investments

An important goal from an investment portfolio standpoint is to emphasize tax efficiency, which entails both tax location and tax-preferential strategies. In the case of tax location, there are a couple of concepts to remember: (1) try to invest in qualified plans (IRA, 401[k], and so forth) for assets that generate interest and dividends taxed at ordinary income tax rates, and (2) emphasize investing in personal accounts for assets with capital gains or preferential tax treatment. When it comes to tax-preferential strategies, assets, including permanent life insurance, real estate, and municipal bonds, could all come into play.

Having the correct tax location for investments often is advantageous. Physicians tend to be in the highest tax bracket and most probably are not living off their portfolio on a day-to-day basis. So, if an investment is generating a 4% taxable dividend and it appears on the tax return, then ordinary income taxes are being paid on money that is remaining in the investment portfolio and not being used for living expenses. At an effective income tax rate of 45% (federal and state), the net earnings on a 4% return are effectively only 2.2%.

My clients have various investment strategies that generate interest and dividend income, which are taxable as ordinary income. These include corporate bonds, real estate investment trusts, senior secured collateralized lending strategies, mutual funds, and so forth. If a client has IRA accounts, it typically makes sense to position these investments within them because all of that interest and dividend income continue to grow tax deferred in the account, rather than being taxed today as ordinary income.

Other investment strategies offer tax benefits as well. These include municipal bonds that generate tax-free income and real estate strategies that can provide depreciation and tax-deferral / opportunities. Additionally, there are stocks/exchange-traded funds (ETFs) that typically generate long-term capital gains when sold, and these rates currently are lower than ordinary income rates. Whenever possible, structuring these investments within the personal, nonpension accounts of clients is an advisable strategy.

### Be Aware of Alternatives

Interest rates are the lowest they have been in decades, leading to extensive news coverage about how fixed-income securities, such as bonds, can be expected to deliver much lower returns for the next 10 years.

As detailed briefly previously, permanent life insurance can offer a beneficial complement to a fixed-income portfolio on a tax-preferential basis. The cash value within these permanent policies can grow tax deferred. If structured properly, such a policy also can generate tax-free distributions during retirement.

There are countless ways to structure a permanent insurance portfolio, with dozens of companies/products/options to choose from. It is important to research all available options and ensure that counsel is independent and objective from an advisor who has experience with and expertise in these strategies. Because of the complexity and potentially significant advantages involved, I take clients through a thorough analysis detailing all of their options as well as the associated costs and benefits.

### PILLAR 3: GROWING WEALTH
*Control What Is Possible and Recognize What Is Not*

No one can precisely predict the day-to-day variations of the stock market, but decades of data prove that staying invested over a long time period should provide positive results. The key to long-term success is managing what is controllable and not diverting resources to what is not. A few examples include the following:

1. Keep investment expenses as low as possible. Investors may elect to take advantage of low-cost, passively managed ETFs, in particular those tracking broad indexes (eg, S&P 500). Data have shown that over long time periods, many actively managed funds fail to outperform their indexes, which can make it difficult to justify their higher internal expenses.[3] On the other hand, some actively managed funds in less-efficient sectors (small cap companies, international/emerging markets, real estate, alternative fixed income, and so forth) have demonstrated a better ability to outperform their indexes. For these reasons, when structuring client portfolios, I tend to allocate 60% to 70% in low-cost indexing strategies to track the broad markets at a very low cost, with the balance in more actively managed and alternative strategies in less-efficient sectors.

2. Maintain a proper allocation among various investment opportunities. Most retail investors typically are invested in US equities, international equities, and fixed income. But well-respected endowments (Yale, Harvard, and so forth)[4] often have much more diversified portfolios that include real estate, hedging strategies, commodities, alternative lending/credit strategies, and so forth. These also can be useful allocations within a personal portfolio, and suitable investments are available with appropriate due diligence.

3. Continually evaluate risk tolerance, goals, and objectives at least annually and rebalance the portfolio accordingly.

A professionally designed portfolio takes these aspects into account and is reviewed and adjusted on an ongoing basis. Often, such portfolios are described as 80/20 or 40/60, where the first number is the percentage of the portfolio invested into equities and the second is the percentage invested into fixed income. Typically, the equities portion of the portfolio grows (or declines) in value faster than the fixed-income portion. During a bull market, a portfolio that originally was designed to be 60/40 might tilt closer to 80/20, as market growth outstrips fixed-income growth. If a market downturn hits at this point, the investor experiences greater losses than planned since 80% of their portfolio is now subjected to equity risk rather than the originally allocated 60%. Conversely, if the initial portfolio investment occurred just prior to a bear market, the portfolio might veer toward 40/60. In this scenario, only 40% of the investor's portfolio would then participate in the subsequent equity market recovery rather than the originally allocated 60%. Regular rebalancing can ensure that investors participate in market fluctuations to the extent suggested by their risk tolerance, goals, and objectives. To ensure portfolios are being properly designed and rebalanced, I take all clients through a comprehensive risk tolerance analysis and match their portfolio with their specific goals and objectives.

### Welcoming the Harvest

Another advisable approach is utilizing tax-loss harvesting strategies for nonqualified accounts.[5] Consider this hypothetical scenario from 2020: in January, an investment account was worth $100,000. Then the steep downturn in March suddenly reduced the account value to $70,000. By November, the market had recovered and the account value returned to $100,000.

If that portfolio was being actively managed for tax-loss harvesting, the managers would have sought opportunities to make trades and capture part of that tax-deductible $30,000 loss before the market recovered. In the process, they would have simultaneously attempted to replace those assets with similar investments.

In the absence of these measures, because the dollar amount in September matched the amount from January, no value would have been created for this account due to the downturn. But if the tax-loss harvesting transactions occurred, the account holder would be able to claim a $30,000 loss to offset taxable gains potentially realized during the year.

### Every Little Bit Helps: Economic Benefits for Families with Children

For single-filing taxpayers who earn less than $139,000 annually,[6] another effective wealth-accumulation strategy is contributing to a Roth IRA. The current annual contribution limit for this vehicle is the lesser amount of $6000 or total earned income.[7] All of the growth within a Roth IRA is completely tax-free, and when the account is accessed for income in retirement, distributions also are 100% tax-free.

For anyone who has teenage children with summer jobs or who are in college with paid internships, utilizing a Roth strategy can be beneficial. If the child receives a W-2 for $6000, why not set up a Roth IRA in his or her name? He or she likely is more interested in spending the hard-earned money on desired items rather than putting it toward a retirement that could be 60 years away, and that perspective certainly is understandable. But there is nothing to stop a parent from gifting a $6000 annual contribution on the child's behalf.

This strategy can be continued for as long as a child is earning income less than $139,000 a year. If that income scenario exists from ages 15 through 30, a total of $90,000 in deposits could grow 100% tax-free for several decades. Assuming a 5% annualized rate of return, by the time the then-adult reaches age 65, that money would amount to more than $1,250,000, completely tax-free under current law. So, an investment strategy that might not seem very impactful today can yield significant wealth in the future.

### Pay for College with Tax-Free Dollars

Speaking about planning and children, 529 plans are a great vehicle to leverage because the earnings are 100% tax-free if utilized for qualified educational expenses. When funding a college education, it always is better to start saving sooner rather than later. Early investment in a 529 plan could see $100,000 grow to $150,000; that extra $50,000 literally is free money for tuition and other related expenses. Alternatively, if those funds were contributed to a conventional investment account, that $50,000 is subject to capital gains and/or ordinary income taxes depending on the tax treatment of the investment gains.

I conduct a college funding analysis with all clients who have children, so they know how much money eventually will be needed as well as the monthly contribution amounts necessary to achieve that goal. Committing to an automatic monthly deposit, no matter how small, is a good practice when beginning this process. As discussed previously regarding retirement contributions, when the money comes out of a bank account every month, it somehow is never missed.

### A GOAL WITHOUT A PLAN IS SIMPLY A WISH

Although this article stresses the importance of 3 basic pillars, the capstone is creating a financial plan. Whether designed by a financial professional or personally, having a plan is of paramount importance. It is impossible to make accurate financial projections for the future without an understanding of what that future should be; the more practical decisions of what is the fastest and/or safest route to get there then can be answered.

Often, new clients present with what can be called piecemeal planning. When they need a will, they find an attorney. When they need insurance, they find an insurance agent. And when they need tax work, they find an accountant. Although each professional may be an expert in his or her field, that expertise addresses only 1 specific need of the client.

Physicians understand how treating 1 medical condition as a standalone issue can be risky. A broad medical, surgical, family, and medication history are among the first questions asked by all health professionals. After the initial evaluation, additional tests may be ordered as well as consultation with other professionals, as appropriate. Once the evaluation is complete, an ideal treatment plan emphasizes a holistic approach, considering the patient's overall health and any possible comorbidities.

An appropriate financial plan follows a similar rubric, promoting overall financial security and simultaneously balancing needs and resources. Financial advisors, regardless of their expertise, need to assess a client's overall financial life or else risk missing an opportunity to create a holistic plan that maximizes benefits in all areas (**Fig. 1**).

### Avoiding Common Errors

As a financial advisor for almost 3 decades, I have seen many common pitfalls[8] within physicians' financial plans. These include

1. Failing to act. Long hours, family commitments, work pressure, and caring for patients all can make it difficult to find time to plan financial health and security. Critical decisions to design and implement strategies can easily be put off for weeks, months, or even years. Albert Einstein once said, "Compound interest is the most powerful force in the universe."[9] Delaying investment decisions results in lost time, which minimizes this important benefit. One of the greatest values an advisor can provide is being proactive about bringing strategies to the attention of clients and then diligently following-up to ensure time is scheduled to discuss and properly implement them.
2. Attempting to time the market. This rarely is a successful strategy and can yield disastrous results (**Fig. 2**). Attempts to time the market

are based on guessing when to sell holdings ahead of a potential downturn and then when to buy back in ahead of a possible climb. Despite the poor odds, many investors try to pull it off. The problem is that the timing must be exactly right not just once (when to sell) but twice (when to buy back in). I have come across situations where someone made the "right" decision to go to cash, but then the stock market recovered 5%, 10%, or 20%, and the person decided it was not time to get back in yet. Suddenly, 6 months or a year passed by and that investor completely missed the rebound.

3. Not considering tax consequences. This pitfall certainly is understandable, considering how complicated and ever-changing tax law can be. When working with a new client, one of the most common missteps I discover is that the investment portfolio was structured with seemingly little attention to proper tax planning. As a result, the client unknowingly was paying additional taxes for years that could have been avoided with appropriate portfolio design and implementation.
4. Lack of proper planning and ongoing review. Every surgeon has a plan in place before entering an operating room. There are not only clear courses of action but also contingency plans for the unexpected. Such careful preparation ensures the best possible outcome for each patient. Unfortunately, the same diligence and care often are not applied by physicians to their personal financial health and well-being. Take the time to clearly define long and short-term goals and objectives. Create a plan and continually review it to ensure proper adjustments are made based on evolving environments. Without a plan, the best possible results never will be achieved.

### "You Don't Know What You Don't Know"

In addition to physicians, I work with many business owner/entrepreneur clients. The most successful of them have an important trait in common—they find the time and allocate the money to work with various coaches/strategists. These specialists help the entrepreneurs constantly grow and improve their businesses while also making them aware of all their options and opportunities.

Many top athletes also use private coaches to improve their skills and success. I work with coaches as well, in both my personal life and professional practice. Through the years, these professionals have helped me implement many

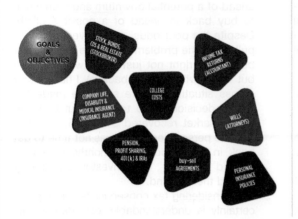 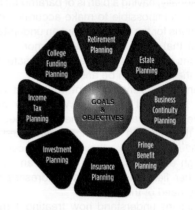

**Fig. 1.** This graphic illustrates a comparison of 2 different methods of financial planning: a piecemeal financial approach *(left)* which utilizes separate resources for each area of financial planning (ie, an accountant for taxes, an attorney for a will, and a stockbroker for investments), and a coordinated financial planning approach *(right)* that unites all areas of financial planning via a comprehensive financial plan led by a financial advisor. Utilizing a financial advisor streamlines all aspects of financial planning and ensures each segment is working in unison toward an investor's financial goals.

beneficial strategies that I had no previous awareness about. It calls to mind the insightful adage, "You don't know what you don't know."

Busy clinicians cannot possibly find the time to identify, research and fully comprehend every potentially beneficial legal/tax/financial strategy available. This is where developing a relationship with an independent, expert advisor who works for a firm with the capabilities to evaluate these strategies; ideally, a long-term relationship between client and advisor results in more perfect knowledge and trust, both of which are beneficial in financial planning.

The alternative can be perilous. I have come across new physician clients in their 50s and 60s and seen the devastating financial scenarios caused by them never putting plans in place or

not properly reviewing and adjusting plans over time. In some cases, physicians can be their own worst enemies regarding financial health—perhaps partly due to their significant education, expertise, and insight. When presented with a strategy, they may feel compelled to analyze it repeatedly, to the point of never making a decision or doing so long after it would have been most advantageous.

Time unfortunately is something that never can be recovered, and the same is true for lost benefits related to compound growth, tax deferral, and tax reduction. When prostate cancer is diagnosed early, at the localized or regional stage, the 5-year relative survival rate is nearly 100%.[10] Similarly, early action can help ensure effective financial planning. Take the time to create a financial

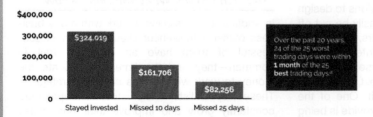

**Fig. 2.** Impact on a $100,000 portfolio of missing the market's best days. This chart shows an analysis of investors' behavior over the past 20 years and how it had an impact on their investment return. Investors who kept their $100,000 investment in the stock market consistently throughout the past 20 years saw the highest portfolio return. Investors who missed out on the top-10 performing days cut gains on their $100,000 investment by nearly half, whereas investors who missed out on the top-25 performing days cut gains on their $100,000 investment by nearly 75%. [a]The only period without a corresponding best day within 1 month was September 17, 2001. Past performance does not guarantee or indicate future results. (*Data from* BlackRock; Bloomberg. Morningstar as of 2/28/20. U.S. stocks are represented by the S&P 500 Index, an unmanaged index that is generally considered representative of the U.S. stock market. Index performance for illustrative purposes only. It is not possible to invest directly in an index.)

plan sooner rather than later and review it often—with this strategy, the odds of success increase exponentially. So, whether as an individual or in partnership with an advisor, taking action is essential and there is no better time than now.

## DISCLOSURE

Christopher Stappas, J.D., CFP®, is a private wealth advisor with 29 years of industry experience. He provides comprehensive advisory services and financial planning to an affluent clientele through Summit Financial LLC, an SEC Registered Investment Adviser and independent advisory firm. Securities brokerage offered through Purshe Kaplan Sterling Investments, Member FINRA/SIPC. Headquartered at 80 State Street, Albany NY 12207 ("PKS"). PKS and Summit Financial, LLC are not affiliated companies. Insurance is offered through Summit Risk Management, LLC, an affiliate of Summit Financial LLC. Past performance is no guarantee of future results. Diversification/asset allocation does not ensure a profit or guarantee against a loss. None of the statements in this article are intended to recommend any security, service, or product or to provide investment, tax or other advice. The views and opinions expressed in this post are solely those of the author and do not represent those of, nor should they be attributed to, Summit Financial LLC and its affiliates. Chris can be reached by email at cstappas@sfr1.com or by phone at 973-292-5432. 10302020-1185.

## REFERENCES

1. Ahmad FA, White AJ, Hiller KM, et al. An assessment of residents' and fellows' personal finance literacy: an unmet medical education need. Int J Med Educ 2017;8:192–204.

2. Retirement topics - 401(k) and profit-sharing plan contribution limits. Internal revenue service. Available at: https://www.irs.gov/retirement-plans/plan-participant-employee/retirement-topics-401k-and-profit-sharing-plan-contribution-limits. Accessed October 29, 2020.

3. Carrel L. Passive management marks decade of beating active U.S. stock funds. Forbes. 2020. Available at: https://www.forbes.com/sites/lcarrel/2020/04/20/passive-beats-active-large-cap-funds-10-years-in-a-row/. Accessed October 29, 2020.

4. Endowment reports. Yale investments office. 2020. Available at: http://investments.yale.edu/reports. Accessed October 29, 2020.

5. Kopp CM. Using tax-loss harvesting to improve investment returns. Investopedia. 2020. Available at: https://www.investopedia.com/articles/taxes/08/tax-loss-harvesting.asp. Accessed October 29, 2020.

6. Amount of Roth IRA contributions that you can make for 2020. Internal Revenue Service. Available at: https://www.irs.gov/retirement-plans/plan-participant-employee/amount-of-roth-ira-contributions-that-you-can-make-for-2020. Accessed October 29, 2020.

7. Retirement topics - IRA contribution limits. Internal revenue service. Available at: https://www.irs.gov/retirement-plans/plan-participant-employee/retirement-topics-ira-contribution-limits. Accessed October 29, 2020.

8. Summit Financial Investment Team. A lesson in behavioral pillars. Summit Financial 2020.

9. Albert Einstein - compound interest. QuotesOnFinance.com. Available at: https://quotesonfinance.com/quote/79/albert-einstein-compound-interest. Accessed October 29, 2020.

10. Survival rates for prostate cancer. American Cancer Society. Available at: https://www.cancer.org/cancer/prostate-cancer/detection-diagnosis-staging/survival-rates.html. Accessed October 29, 2020.

# Moving?

## Make sure your subscription moves with you!

To notify us of your new address, find your **Clinics Account Number** (located on your mailing label above your name), and contact customer service at:

**Email: journalscustomerservice-usa@elsevier.com**

**800-654-2452** (subscribers in the U.S. & Canada)
**314-447-8871** (subscribers outside of the U.S. & Canada)

**Fax number: 314-447-8029**

**Elsevier Health Sciences Division**
**Subscription Customer Service**
**3251 Riverport Lane**
**Maryland Heights, MO 63043**

*To ensure uninterrupted delivery of your subscription, please notify us at least 4 weeks in advance of move.

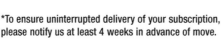

Printed and bound by CPI Group (UK) Ltd, Croydon, CR0 4YY

03/10/2024

01040370-0011